ER: Enter at Your Own Risk

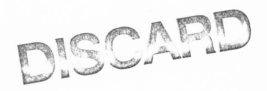

ER: ENTER AT YOUR OWN RISK

How To Avoid Dangers Inside Emergency Rooms

Joel Cohen, M.D.

New Horizon Press
Far Hills, New Jersey

New Horizon Press
P.O. Box 669
Far Hills, NJ 07931

Joel Cohen
    ER: Enter At Your Own Risk
        How to Avoid Dangers Inside Emergency Rooms

Cover Design: Mike Stromberg / The Great American Art Company
Interior Design: Susan M. Sanderson

Library of Congress Control Number: 2001089170

ISBN: 0-88282-205-5
New Horizon Press

Manufactured in the U.S.A.

2005   2004   2003   2002   2001 / 5 4 3 2 1

Dear Tania, Daniel and Andrew:

Grandma Tania watches you
In the park
At the zoo.
Teaching you how best to be,
Having taught her best to me.

The great secret known to internists,
but still hidden from the general public...
is that most things get better by themselves.
Most things, in fact, are better by morning.

Lewis Thomas

The secret of the care of the patient
is in *caring for* the patient.

Dr. Francis Weld Peabody

AUTHOR'S NOTE

In order to protect privacy, fictitious names and identities have been given to some individuals in this book, and otherwise identifying characteristics have been altered. For the purposes of simplifying usage, the pronouns his/him and her are often used interchangeably.

Any medical advice in this book serves only as a supplement to, not a substitute for, a physical examination, medical history and needed lab tests performed by your licensed healthcare provider.

TABLE OF CONTENTS

PREFACE

Hang the smoke detectors. Map out a fire drill. You do not chance a fire ravaging your home and your precious loved ones. You even write out a last will and testament to plan for the unexpected. But have you thought about which hospital emergency room to go to for a heart attack or broken limb? What would you do if a child became seriously ill or began convulsing because of a burning fever? The chances for sudden illness to strike are greater than for a house fire to occur yet most people do little to plan for medical calamities.

Advance planning is crucial if you want solid medical care for sudden sickness. You develop crushing chest pain, for example. Which nearby hospital ER has the best capabilities to save your life and which hospital ER might be ineffective in treating your massive heart attack? Up to one-third of heart attacks do not even cause chest pain. Do you know the less common symptoms of a heart attack? Do you know how to choose the best emergency care facility for your particular problem? The answers to these questions may very well save your life.

If your child becomes drowsy and spikes a 105-degree temperature can all hospital emergency rooms provide equally good care? You slice your hand with a kitchen knife. Can you avoid the long wait and havoc of the emergency room and get quality care elsewhere? Few people plan how and where to seek urgent medical care, yet careful pre-planning might prolong your life and health as well as that of your loved ones.

Answering these key questions before you fall ill can help both you and healthcare professionals avoid mistakes. Planning ahead can also save you money and help to avoid inconvenience. Why should a young, healthy person prepare in advance for serious illness? Preparation is important for everybody, not just the frail and elderly. A healthy child can suffer an appendicitis attack. An athlete can smash bones and skull in a car accident. And even a doctor can take a spill.

Three years ago, I fell off a ladder while cleaning leaves from the gutter on my house. As the ladder slid back, I came crashing to the ground while desperately clutching the top end. With the force of my eleven-foot descent, my chest slammed into and actually dented a rung of the forged aluminum ladder. It felt like a sledgehammer slamming my chest. I soon felt dizzy and disoriented and had the frightening thought that I might be hemorrhaging from a torn heart artery in my chest. My wife saw me on the ground and quickly called the paramedics' number that was posted near our telephone. Soon after they arrived I was able to stand up and talk. I agreed with the paramedics that I should get checked out at the local hospital ER, but did not need to go to a trauma center that was a thirty-minute drive away. At that moment, I was thankful that I had taken the time to visit and evaluate the hospital and its emergency care facility when we had first moved into the neighborhood. I was already confident that they provided quality emergency medical assistance. As I expected, I was well taken care of at the local hospital. My tests were normal, and I went home having learned two valuable lessons: medical emergencies are almost always sudden and not the time to be trying to decide which emergency care facility is best and...hire someone to clean the gutters.

Develop a solid plan of action *now*. You do not want to make key healthcare decisions in a cloud of panic during a crisis. With nearly one hundred million annual emergency room visits in this country, nobody is immune to unexpected illness or injury. Sooner or later, you or your loved one will end up prone and vulnerable on a hard stretcher, subject to doctors and medical personnel you know nothing about.

How can this book help? Think of the emergency room as a dense, foreboding jungle. This book serves as guide and map to sidestep dangers and lead you safely through. Is seeking emergency care really like walking through a treacherous jungle? Yes, unfortunately, emergency room care has become unreliable and unpredictable—even hazardous! While emergency rooms usually help patients and save lives, they have become fertile ground for avoidable medical mistakes and tragedies.

ER: Enter At Your Own Risk provides an insider's tour of the chaotic ER with an experienced emergency care physician as your guide. This book can help you sidestep trouble and danger by planning ahead. It is chock full of key advice for properly managing sudden illnesses that might strike you, your child, a spouse or frail parent. Leave *ER: Enter At Your Own Risk* on your coffee table. Refer to it from time to time. This resource can help you plan wisely, stay informed, sensibly manage minor emergencies and properly evaluate and use emergency care facilities. Read on and find out how to get healed, not harmed by emergency medical care.

1

PATIENTS' HORROR STORIES FROM WITHIN A TROUBLED SYSTEM

Emergency care system, heal thyself. Our nation's emergency care system is troubled, but the band-aid approach to cure the problems will not work. Problems within the current system tunnel far deeper than having a few inept doctors and nurses working in hospital emergency rooms. Horror stories of poor treatment and indifferent care are no longer oddities. They have become routine, daily occurrences. The public regularly learns of these grim stories from newspaper and television reports and shakes its collective head, grateful not to be involved in such medical mishaps. But any of us could be the victim of a hectic and hazardous emergency room and its highly stressed staff. Consider that each time a medical horror story appears in the news, there are countless other unnoticed tragedies happening everyday. These silent stories won't make the news, but still cause individuals pain, disability and even death. Sadly, most of these people will never find out that their suffering could have been avoided.

In our current healthcare system, the law of supply and demand for emergency room care has gone askew. Each year, a tidal wave of nearly one hundred million patients comes crashing through hospital emergency room doors, while budget cuts have trimmed to the bare bones physician and nurse staffing. Why are so many patients overburdening our emergency departments? Societal trends, physician practice patterns, hospital or emergency department closings, seasonal epidemics and a modern plague all play a role.

The consequences of emergency room overcrowding are obvious. What does any worker do when they have work assignments that should be handled by two people? They cut corners, rush through things and make mistakes. At best, they do mediocre work on some projects; at worst, they do a lousy job. There are also times when excessive stress and demands lead to apathy and hostility. The worker simply does not care anymore. This is a scary thought when those extra "projects" are patients and the workers are medical professionals. Overcrowding in the ER inevitably leads to medical mistakes, miscommunications, errors in judgment, prolonged pain and suffering and even death.

The true patient experiences that follow are meant to open eyes and evoke constructive emotional responses. Similar tragedies are daily occurrences in emergency departments across the country—only most go unnoticed and unpublicized. These true stories serve to inform you about a terribly disturbing truth: tragedies and mistakes beyond your wildest imagination *can* and *do* occur in busy, over-burdened emergency departments. Chaos promotes calamity. Becoming an informed patient, however, can help to deter bad ER experiences. People must learn about the flaws in the emergency care system so they are better positioned to guard against the dangers yet take advantage of all it has to offer. Some underlying problems that promote errors in emergency rooms are systemic—the entire process of providing healthcare must be overhauled to improve patient care and safety. Do not believe for a moment that the prestigious hospital nearby or the quiet community hospital down the road is an exception. Horror stories happen everywhere.

Ignoring the failings of our emergency care system—claiming it does not apply to you, because you are healthy or careful or smart—is taking a huge gamble. Auto accidents happen everyday, people slip on ice covered sidewalks, ingest toxic substances, slide into home plate at the wrong angle, etc., etc. Injuries and accidents are always unplanned emergencies. Do you have any medical illnesses that can become an emergency? Does a parent or child have such an illness, like asthma or heart problems? Even if you or your children and other loved ones are healthy, this is the time to map out a strategy for unexpected illness or injury and to practice prevention. Educate yourself. Call local hospitals to learn about the level of emergency care services they provide. Ask how many doctors they have working each shift in the ER. Does the emergency room use physician assistants or nurse practitioners? Stop by and look over local urgent care facilities. Ask neighbors for recommendations. Do advance planning. Ask your doctor questions. Be proactive with your own care or the care of a loved one. Do not allow yourself to become an ER horror tale as the next three patients did.

THREE HORROR STORIES

Patricia's Suffering

Patricia's scream reverberated across the emergency room. Doctors, nurses and patients stared in eerie silence. From behind a blue curtain, Patricia had just learned emergency rooms sometimes provide the worst of care. Horror stories in newspapers about shoddy emergency care did not shake Patricia's belief that emergency rooms healed patients and saved lives. Perhaps she had been wrong.

Just a few hours earlier Patricia was working at her desk when she felt a soaking wet gush. She had heard stories of harmless bleeding during early pregnancy, but something wasn't right. She became light-headed and soon found herself in an unfamiliar emergency room with an intravenous line in her arm.

The emergency room doctor entered the room and wondered if Patricia's pale face betrayed a hidden illness or if she was simply fair-skinned. Her pulse rate was one hundred beats per minute. Was it anxiety or hidden blood loss that caused her rapid heartbeat? Her normal blood pressure of "one hundred over seventy" provided some reassurance.

The nurse gave Patricia a reassuring smile at the start of the internal examination. The physician inserted the speculum and saw large blood clots inside. He told Patricia she might be having a miscarriage and she tearfully confided her concerns about losing her baby. She was distraught over the possibility of this loss, but her immediate worry was being at an unfamiliar place with unknown doctors one hour away from her gynecologist's hospital. The nurse and doctor assuaged her fears and promised to take good care of her.

The doctor and nurse left the room and exchanged worried glances. They knew Patricia would have to stay in the hospital for observation. The pale face, rapid heartbeat, dizziness and heavy bleeding forebode a more serious problem.

While waiting for the on-call gynecologist to arrive, there was a frantic call for help from the "GYN" room. Patricia's blood pressure had plummeted and death loomed near as she hemorrhaged from a complication of a miscarriage.

The emergency room doctor started a second intravenous line and her condition stabilized by the time the on-call specialist arrived. The gynecologist closed the curtain to examine Patricia. Moments later, that chilling scream of cutting pain silenced the entire emergency department. The ER doctor wondered what had happened. He inched toward the curtain.

A pale-faced nurse emerged from behind the curtain with a bloody, dead fetus in her trembling hand. The nurse described how the gynecologist stuck his hand up Patricia's vaginal canal then into her uterus and, like a dentist pulling out a deeply imbedded wisdom tooth, yanked out the dead fetus. There was no warning, no anesthesia and no compassion. Patricia later went to the operating room for scraping of the uterus, a procedure that made this brutal experience unnecessary.

Patricia was a victim of shoddy emergency care, because one link in the chain of her care proved faulty—a specialist with less than special care-taking capabilities. Patricia was subjected to intense suffering, both physical and emotional, and possible long-term harm that could have been easily avoided.

Liz's Misdiagnosis

Liz awoke one morning and felt pain in her upper back. *Must have slept wrong*, she thought. But the pain didn't go away with over-the-counter medicine or time. A while later she became aware of her difficulty breathing. It felt labored, as if each breath was an effort. Liz's keen instincts led her to seek care at a trusted community urgent care facility. The doctor and nurse who evaluated her found her blood pressure to be extremely high. Perhaps her blood pressure was high because she was in pain? The experienced physician was puzzled. This woman seemed more likely to ignore her health than to baby it, the doctor reasoned. Yet she sought medical care for back pain without sustaining an injury. It did not add up. On the hunch this might be an unusual case of a more ominous problem, the doctor ordered an electrocardiogram. It proved to be clearly abnormal, but did not conclusively show a heart attack.

After giving Liz appropriate medication, the nurse called an ambulance to transport her to a hospital emergency room. Liz was reluctant to go and had difficulty accepting that, at age fifty, she could be having a heart problem. The doctor wrote up a note for Liz to bring with her indicating a diagnosis of "Angina, rule out myocardial infarction." Liz also had with her a copy of the electrocardiogram with the abnormal interpretation scribbled on top. Before she left, the doctor instructed Liz *not* to let the emergency staff rush her out and not take her seriously. By appearances, she seemed okay. She was neither gasping for air nor writhing in pain. Her skin color was neither healthy bronze nor gray-ish-blue. She appeared calm and in no distress. Appearances, however, can be deceiving. What's more, Liz had experienced less typical symptoms for a possible heart condition, muddying the diagnostic waters. Because Liz was armed with much key information from the first doctor, her diagnosis and treatment should have been simple. But it rarely is.

A short time later a doctor-in-training from the hospital emergency room called the urgent care office to ask if they had Liz's home telephone number. *How odd!* the doctor thought. *Since she had left for the emergency room just a short while earlier, couldn't they simply ask her for her number?* The doctor grew concerned that perhaps something had happened to Liz or that she never got to the emergency department.

What had happened was that Liz was discharged from the ER in under three hours time—unusual even for a minor ailment in a busy emergency room. Clearly, inexperienced and unsupervised doctors-in-training or students evaluated Liz in the emergency room. What was not so clear was how or why they did not take the cues given to them by the first doctor. Perhaps the overwhelmed young doctors ignored the note and electrocardiogram or never checked the emergency room chart for additional information. More importantly, why didn't they simply wait to get the blood test results back, which would have indicated whether or not Liz had suffered a heart attack, before discharging her? There was little doubt Liz was more than happy to accept the news she could go home with false reassurance that all was fine. Based on how she felt, however, both she and her daughter suspected otherwise.

The blood test results came back positive for heart muscle damage. Liz had suffered a heart attack without experiencing chest pain! Studies have found that as many as one in three heart attacks do *not* involve chest pain. Furthermore, heart attack sufferers who do not have the classic symptoms as publicized in the news or depicted on television (i.e., crushing chest pain, collapse) are more likely to delay seeking care. Heart attack sufferers with less typical symptoms also get fewer appropriate treatments and have a greater likelihood of dying in the hospital.

In fact, for every one hundred heart attack sufferers, about four or five will be mistakenly sent home from the emergency room. Those who are sent home have significantly more complications—including death—than those properly diagnosed, according to medical studies. Liz was lucky and once she was informed by the hospital ER that her test had come back positive for heart damage, she sought treatment and made a successful recovery.

Alexis's Tragedy

The following tragic story is an excerpt from an article originally printed in the *Boston Globe*.[1] Titled "Patients at Risk: Hospital Errors," the award-winning work illustrates just how powerful and painful deadly hospital mistakes can be.

Alexis Masiello was going to go home.

After spending her entire two and a half years in hospitals undergoing a dozen operations to repair birth defects in her chest and stomach, after thousands of hours of therapy and meals delivered by drip, the chocolate-haired toddler was at last going home. Her father had quit his job to take care of her, her mother was putting the finishing touches on her bedroom.

But on the night of October 10, 1996, the medical system at Franciscan Children's Hospital in Brighton that had kept Alexis alive failed her. Sometime after 7:30 her breathing tube became disconnected. Alarms should have sounded, and may have, but no one came. The licensed practical nurse assigned to Alexis was meeting with an insurance executive. A childcare worker eventually noticed warning lights on a TV monitor, but it was too late. By then, Alexis's brain had been robbed of oxygen for too long.

Two days later Alexis Masiello died, without ever making it home.

Michele Masiello drew into herself after the death of her daughter Alexis. She'd already been stretched by the demands of three children at home in Oxford and one in the hospital in Brighton, a divorce and remarriage, and her job as a paralegal. One steamy day in July she swallowed several fistfuls of pills, then was taken by ambulance to Worcester's Memorial Hospital.

Again, things went wrong. Nurses gave her medicine to calm her. When that didn't work they restrained her, then apparently left her unattended. Sometime over the next ninety minutes she coughed up and inhaled the powder they'd given her to absorb the overdosed drugs. This blocked her airway. By the time nurses checked on her she'd stopped breathing.

Michele died ten days later, nine months to the day after her daughter.

The Masiello cases are more than isolated tragedies. They are a lens into the unsettling and unseen world of medication errors, faulty diagnoses, delays in treatment and other preventable mistakes in hospitals.

These true experiences are a small sampling of what can and does happen in our nation's emergency departments. Key factors underlying these medical miscues are emergency room overcrowding and under-staffing. Teaching and big city hospital emergency departments are hardest hit by overcrowding, but community and suburban hospitals also are very much affected. A community hospital might see far fewer patients, but they make up for it by having considerably less staff to care for those patients. Overcrowding leads to lack of supervision, chaos, confusion and, ultimately, tragic mistakes.

OVERCROWDING

What exactly is emergency room overcrowding? The answer might seem obvious, but there are many different definitions. Is overcrowding defined by a long patient wait to be treated? Are patients who are admitted into the hospital but held in the emergency room waiting for a bed counted? Does the criteria apply to patients who are brought into the main emergency area quickly, but are not properly evaluated for many minutes or hours? Is it the many patients who are cheated of privacy, basic peace and quiet when they are interviewed, examined and kept in a hallway? Is one or all of these overcrowding?

Dr. Arthur Kellerman, an emergency room director, points out an interesting definition of overcrowding in an editorial he wrote, which was published in the journal, *Annals of Emergency Medicine*: "I suspect most emergency department directors would give the same response provided by a Supreme Court justice who was asked to define obscene material—'I know it when it see it.'"[2] Drs. Robert Derlet and John Richards, in a January 2000 *Annals of Emergency Medicine* article, offer what is perhaps the best definition of overcrowding in the emergency room: when nurses and doctors feel rushed to the point that they believe quality of care is compromised.[3]

It seems, on the surface, that we are all simply victims of too much demand for care in a society where everyone seems to believe all health problems are urgent and must be tended to immediately. Does this mean everyone should just learn to live (or die) with an overtaxed emergency care system? Or do we need to work to make changes in how emergency care is given and how it is utilized? This would seem to be, but it is not necessarily the case. There are those who do not want to change the system and remedy overcrowding, according to Drs. Derlet and Richards. In their reply to a letter to the editor in *Annals of Emergency Medicine*, they reveal several shocking controversies.[4] One suggested dilemma they address is "the reluctance of certain hospitals to make any effort to fix the problem" of overcrowded and chaotic ERs. Some hospitals consider the emergency department to be a "gateway for the uninsured." These hospitals have no interest in expanding staffs and facilities of their emergency rooms out of fear that more capacity will attract more indigent, nonpaying patients. According to Derlet and Richards, keeping ERs overcrowded serves as a repellent to all but the sickest patients who have no choice other than to seek emergency treatment.[5]

As to why so many patients are overburdening our emergency care system, there are several major and a few minor factors. The major reasons can be categorized into sicker patients, more patients and no other places for patients to go.

Sicker Patients

Increased violence with guns and knives as well as more widespread drug abuse have led to a deluge of critically injured, strung-out or drug-overdosed people burdening our emergency care facilities. Sadly, it is not rare to see scenes like that of four gunshot victims lying on stretchers for hours without treatment at an inner-city hospital in Los Angeles.[6]

The growing elderly population often suffer from chronic and debilitating diseases that frequently land them in emergency rooms. In addition, many nursing home patients do not get the close medical supervision they need. They can be seriously ill by the time they are sent to an emergency room. On the other end of the spectrum, some nursing home patients are rushed to an emergency room for a slight fever or cough before the responsible physician thoroughly evaluates them at the nursing home.

The AIDS epidemic can be likened to a modern plague and is another cause for sicker emergency room patients. These afflicted patients frequent emergency rooms with serious and puzzling illnesses, requiring a great deal of nurse and physician time. AIDS has also contributed to a resurgence of tuberculosis, a serious and contagious lung and body infection that requires patient isolation. Until tuberculosis is suspected or diagnosed and the patient isolated, the disease can be transmitted to staff and other patients. If this situation mushrooms, it will place further strain on the emergency care system.

More Patients

If more seriously injured and sicker patients are not taxing enough, spiraling healthcare costs have also taken their toll by leading more people to seek emergency room care as their first and only option. Over forty million Americans have no health insurance, because it is unaffordable to individuals or small businesses. Furthermore, many doctors will not see welfare patients in their office since welfare payments to doctors barely cover paperwork costs.

Since 1994 over 340 hospitals or emergency departments have shut their doors, according to reports by the American Hospital Association and the Office of the Inspector General. These changes were the result of hospital mergers and budget cuts. The math is simple. More patients going to fewer hospital emergency departments equals overcrowding.

Medical practice patterns have also changed dramatically, but not for the better. Change began with the extinction of the family, house-call-making doctor. Some vestiges of this rare breed remain, but few modern doctors make house calls. To take it one step further, few doctors today are readily available for their patients. Primary care doctors can be virtually impossible to see on urgent notice. When a sudden injury or illness strikes or a patient's condition worsens, many physicians send their patients to be evaluated by "strangers" at an emergency room rather than try to work the patients into their crowded appointment schedules. With this approach, the family physician need not interrupt busy office hours or his or her personal life. In today's practices, there are usually "covering" or back-up doctors at night who will send patients to an emergency room to get treatment. It is, unfortunately, sometimes easier for doctors to have others care for and evaluate their patients.

Doctor availability dilemmas grow more complex. Many doctors are unable to give their patients more personal attention, because in these days of managed healthcare, they must see forty to sixty patients each day just to make ends meet. There is also a shortage of primary care physicians, because specialization has become the only way to earn large salaries in medicine. A one-hour history and physical earns perhaps $150; a one-hour procedure like colonoscopy or surgery earns hundreds to thousands of dollars. Fewer primary care doctors means lengthy appointment delays and less access to preventive care. Patients who fall ill are often told there are no appointments for days to weeks in advance. Sadly, few patients get to know those primary care doctors who do exist, because, in many cases, people must change primary care doctors each time they change insurance coverage or jobs. Where do these people go for more immediate care? They turn to emergency rooms, the patient safety net.

Seasonal epidemics such as influenza (the flu) can devastate already overwhelmed emergency rooms across the country. Some good advice:

If possible, avoid emergency rooms during the winter cold and flu seasons. Patients might have to wait many hours before they are seen by doctors or nurses and can even catch a cold or flu while in the waiting room. If winter is the season to avoid, Mondays and Friday or Saturday nights are the days to avoid, if at all possible, due to predictably higher patient volume.

No Place For Patients To Go

A major cause for ER backlog that commonly gets mentioned is the fact that hospitals do not have enough beds in intensive care, heart-monitoring units and regular medical and surgical floors to allow patient flow out from emergency room hallways and into regular hospital rooms. Several related issues do not get as much focus and are kept hushed. For instance, many hospitals have entire wards filled with unused beds, but financial constraints do not allow these wards to remain staffed and operational. Drs. Derlet and Richard also point out in their article that they have personally toured several "full" hospitals. They discovered, in fact, that wards were empty or hospital beds were reserved for paying patients to be admitted.[7] It is not uncommon for hospital wards to "conceal" available beds in order to delay another admission from the emergency room and the extra work that ensues.

Another key factor that keeps emergency rooms in overdrive is "boarding" patients in the ER, as described in a letter to the editor in the journal *Annals of Emergency Medicine*. The emergency room doctor who authored the letter describes how patients are routinely admitted into the hospital yet remain in emergency room hallways rather than hospital rooms. ER nurses must continue to monitor and care for these patients as well as new patients who arrive in the emergency room. Doctors on the ward are responsible for overseeing such patients' care and might check on them just a few minutes each day. "Boarding" saves hospitals money by eliminating the need to open another ward or expand intensive care beds. "Boarding" also compromises patient care as these very ill patients cannot be watched as closely as they need to be.

High technology such as MRIs or CAT scans and specialized blood tests can help doctors make lifesaving diagnoses in the emergency room. These tests and procedures, however, also hinder the system by causing backlogs in emergency departments. Doctors and patients must wait hours to have these tests performed and to retrieve the results. Precious ER beds remain occupied as the waiting rooms and hallways fill up.

A number of minor factors add to the dangerous overcrowding dilemma in emergency rooms. Emergency staff has a high rate of burnout and turnover. The more experienced professionals leave emergency medicine out of frustration or stress and, frequently, less experienced staff replaces them. The result: less efficiency and professional experience equals lower quality care. A nursing shortage continues to affect many areas and, in fact, hospitals are replacing skilled nurses with less skilled (and less expensive) medical or nurse's assistants.

Money shortages in the healthcare industry have also led to bare minimum staffing of emergency rooms. Teaching hospitals count on using doctors-in-training to augment ER staff, at the cost of having experienced doctors on the front lines of emergency medicine and trauma care. Community hospitals usually have just one and only one doctor per shift. If two seriously ill patients arrive within minutes, one will have to wait minutes to hours for more thorough medical care. What's more, clerical staff has been cut, too. While that may not seem important, it means the doctors and nurses must spend more time on clerical tasks rather than patient care. That slows patient flow further and brings doctors' and nurses' frustrations to their boiling points. Doctors and nurses must also chart many details, not necessarily for the individual patient's benefit, but rather out of fear of potential lawsuits. The result: more unnecessary scribbling on charts, less patient care and greater delays in providing timely and effective medical treatment for the ER patient.

Not surprisingly, a lone doctor working a community hospital emergency room who sees fifty patients in a shift—many that are critically ill—can easily become overwhelmed. At busier university hospitals, the havoc can lead to unsupervised care of patients' serious problems by inexperienced medical students and doctors-in-training. The end result of these forces is an emergency department staff barely keeping its collective head above water. Mistakes are made. Apathy abounds. Healthcare workers ultimately are buried under this unmanageable patient load and thus cannot provide the best care possible for the unsuspecting emergency room patient.

LEAVING WITHOUT BEING SEEN:
A GAPING TEAR IN THE "PATIENT SAFETY NET"

ER overcrowding issues certainly dilute the quality of care patients receive. It is more troubling, however, that emergency rooms were once considered the "patient safety net"—an always reliable haven for medical care—but can no longer be fully relied upon. Large numbers of seriously ill patients are leaving the emergency room without being seen by doctors because they are too sick to sit around and wait. One example of this troubling trend is that of a man with abdominal pain who left a California emergency room without treatment after hours of waiting. He was admitted to another intensive care unit only days later near death from a ruptured spleen.[8] Nearly one in twenty people who sought emergency care in Los Angeles left without being seen by a doctor, according to a study done at the Harbor-UCLA Medical Center. Alarmingly, studies suggest that about half of patients who leave without getting medical care truly require urgent medical evaluation or treatment. One in twenty of these patients need hospital admission within two weeks of leaving crowded emergency rooms.[9] Many patients who leave without being evaluated have nowhere else to turn for medical care. If things get worse, they often will try different emergency rooms, hoping for better care.

Our nation's emergency departments save many lives. Despite this, you place your life and well-being in jeopardy each time you walk through those metal ER doors. Unfortunately, there are no accurate statistics tallied on patient death and harm that could have been avoided with faster or better care. Subtle harm, neglect and oversights often go unmentioned, unnoticed or unattributed. To get excellent emergency care, you must learn how to sidestep and avoid the dangers inherent in all emergency rooms. Only then can you avoid becoming the next ER horror story.

PART

2

THE DANGERS—
AND THEIR SOLUTIONS

The tragic yet avoidable stories you have read about in the previous
section illustrate clearly that dangers abound in emergency rooms.
These horrific experiences, sadly, are not rare exceptions. Before you
rush to seek care at an emergency room, consider these jaw-dropping
facts:

- The large majority of our nation's emergency departments lack the
  most effective treatments for a massive heart attack. A person who
  suffers a major heart attack might die only because he or she went
  to the wrong hospital.
- The emergency room doctor who treats your ailment might be
  inexperienced, inadequately trained and downright unqualified to
  treat your illness.
- Specialist care you receive in an emergency room is as variable as
  the weather. That cardiologist who treats your heart attack or surgeon who removes your appendix might be excellent or inadequate. Emergency room workers usually know which doctors are
  inept, but might feel pressured to put your health in such doctors'
  dangerous hands because of on-call policies.
- The person who first screens your medical problem is often a desk
  clerk with no medical experience or a rushed nurse who hurries
  through a thirty-second screening interview. Either situation can
  lead to medical calamity.
- Your complaint of a wrenched back might buy you a set of unnecessary lower back X rays. The radiation that tunnels through your
  body is roughly equivalent to getting one chest X ray everyday for

an entire year! Many other unnecessary tests and procedures may
be ordered or performed on you in the emergency room.
- About one out of every 100 patients who gets routine clot-dissolving treatment for a heart attack will suffer the dreaded complication—a brain bleed.

A trip to the emergency room without proper information and
preparation can, ironically, prove to be hazardous to your health.

DANGER #1
DOING MORE HARM THAN GOOD

First do no harm. Doctors frequently ignore this basic tenet of the Hippocratic oath, which is a foundation of medical care, but you should not. Harming patients is manifested in three devastating ways in the emergency room (and hospital) setting.

- Treatments that are worse than the disease for which they are given
- Risky or unnecessary tests and procedures
- Outright neglect or costly time delays

TREATMENTS THAT ARE WORSE THAN THE DISEASE

Karen wished she had known sooner about the doctrine of care called *first do no harm.* She and her husband, Bob, assumed people always left the emergency room better off than when they arrived. They found out too late that nothing could be further from the truth.

On this tragic day, Karen learned about harm the hard way. Bob was forty-three years old, had two small children and was too young to die. He lay motionless in the intensive care unit as the priest gave last rites. Karen gazed at her husband and sobbed, her cries drowned out by the hissing ventilator that cyclically inflated his lungs. She could not understand how her companion of thirteen years could suddenly be in a coma. Two days ago Bob was watching a football game when he complained in his husky voice of severe chest pressure and difficulty breathing—but at least he could talk. Now the doctors told Karen her husband was brain dead and would never speak again. "How could my husband wind up this way—all he had was a small heart attack?" she incredulously asked the silent doctors standing around her husband's bed. In the ER, the cardiologist had told Bob and Karen that chances for a serious complication were small. Yet this loving husband and father fell victim to a treatment that proved to be worse than the illness for which it was given.

Bob lay comatose from a brain bleed. He did not fall or get hit over the head. Bob had no puzzling disease. His bleed came as a complication from treatment he received for his mild heart attack. The clot-dissolving drug called tissue plasminogen activator (tPA) breaks apart a clot that is clogging up a heart-feeding artery. In essence, it stops a heart attack in its tracks. This amazing drug, however, can cause bleeding anywhere in the body. Perhaps the cardiologist understated the risks of treatment. The words, "a small chance for a serious bleeding complication" may signify little to an anxious patient and spouse awaiting medical treatment in a bustling ER. In this case, the result of overly aggressive treatment is especially sad, because Bob suffered only a mild heart attack that would not have been debilitating and from which he would have quickly recovered.

Clot-dissolving treatment for a heart attack does lower death and heart failure rates, but a closer look at the statistics can be alarming. For every one hundred patients who receive clot-dissolving treatment, one will suffer the most dreaded and still unpredictable complication—a brain bleed. The elderly are at greatest risk since chances for a brain bleed double in people who are over seventy-five years of age. In fact, recently reported data raised concern that clot-dissolving treatment might cause more deaths (than in untreated patients) in this age group.[1] About two thirds of those who suffer a brain bleed will die from the complication. Even those who avoid a brain bleed, serious bleeding can occur anywhere in the body, often necessitating a blood transfusion.

Bob's wife learned a valuable lesson from this tragedy: ask questions and seriously consider the answers you receive. Sadly, she did not know which questions to ask. Like many people, including some doctors, she believed it is always better to treat, to test and to act rather than to let someone heal with time.

Pill-Popping Predicaments

Many people are relieved when their doctor says, "I'll give you antibiotics just in case," even if the doctor suspects not a bacterial infection, but a viral infection which is unaffected by antibiotics. Patients frequently demand medication, believing pills are a panacea for everything, but doctors who give "just-in-case" treatments are not doing their patients a service. Consider this dramatic scenario that can happen to you or your loved ones:

Tom thought it would be a typical day when he was awakened by the morning sun shining through his window. He was almost dead wrong.

Sitting at the breakfast table, Tom popped an oval antibiotic pill into his mouth and washed down the bitter taste with a few gulps of orange juice. He had just been prescribed a seven-day course of antibiotics for a mild upper respiratory infection. "I have no time to be sick," he had told his doctor. He smacked his lips then buried his nose into the business section of the morning newspaper. Before Tom finished the first article, a hot, flushing sensation flooded his body from head to toes. He felt the room spinning, then a suffocating swelling in his throat. He managed to call out his wife's name before he collapsed onto the tile floor of the kitchen.

Tom's wife found him gasping for air. His face was swollen and fiery red. When the ambulance crew arrived, it was clear to them that he was experiencing an anaphylactic reaction, the most severe type of allergic reaction, to the antibiotic he had just ingested. An adrenaline shot helped to clear the flushing and swelling and Tom survived this potentially deadly reaction to the medication. The doctor who prescribed the antibiotic never told Tom he believed the infection was viral, not bacterial, but instead prescribed the medication to placate Tom. As evidenced by both Bob's and Tom's cases, treatments can clearly prove to be worse than the illness for which they are given.

If you knew a life threatening allergic reaction occurs approximately once in every 1000 uses of penicillin, would you still want antibiotics "just in case?" To look at this in another way, with millions of penicillin prescriptions written each year, thousands of people might experience a bad response or even suffer an anaphylactic reaction and be at risk for death.

Taking the latest antibiotic might sound helpful and reassuring when you have a bad cold, but unexpected and severe reactions to medications can occur in people even after the drug has undergone years of rigorous drug testing. Prescription drugs cause reactions that require hospitalization in 1.5 million people each year and as many as 100,000 of these people die.[2] This puts prescription medication high on the list of causes for death in our country. In fact, over fifty percent of approved drugs cause serious bad reactions, which were not detected prior to government drug approval.[3]

A major pharmaceutical company, for instance, stopped distribution of the antibiotic Omniflox after reports of three deaths and about fifty severe reactions. Omniflox is not an isolated case. The heart medication Flecainide was approved for wide use before further testing revealed more people died when taking the drug than when not using the drug. More recently, weight loss pills may have been associated with serious heart and lung effects, even after many people used them just for casual weight loss. Rezulin, a diabetes drug, was linked to reports of liver damage severe enough to finally have it pulled from the market in the United States in March 2000. A heartburn medicine called Propulsid has been severely restricted in its use due to reports of deaths from heart rhythm disturbances. A vaccine for Rotavirus, which helps to prevent a devastating infection that causes severe diarrhea and vomiting in babies, was recently pulled from the shelves, only weeks after it was approved. Numerous reports of potentially serious intestinal complications in babies who recently got vaccinated were accumulating. The list grows longer and longer. No drug is totally harmless. Unpredictable reactions such as organ damage, rash, throat or tongue swelling, shock and even death are potential dangers from taking any medication.

There is another reason not to use antibiotics needlessly. Unnecessary drug use can have far-reaching detrimental effects on you and society. Each time you take an antibiotic inappropriately, you might be creating a "monster" bacteria inside you that grows resistant to that once useful drug. You may be at risk for severe infection from the now resistant bacteria or you might spread the bug to others. Certain strains of tuberculosis, for example, are now resistant to most medications in our drug arsenal mainly because of misuse of antibiotics. These resistant strains develop into the deadly, untreatable infections we hear about more and more often. Some strains of pneumococcus, the bug that causes most bacterial ear and respiratory infections, have also grown resistant to nearly all antibiotics.

This is why *no* action can at times be wiser than treatment. Many illnesses do get better with time so medication is not always the answer for each and every ailment. The *Physician's Desk Reference* (PDR) lists dozens of side effects for each drug. After scanning the many possible reactions to each medication, you might elect to never again take another pill. Bear in mind, however, while it is foolhardy to demand medication that is unnecessary, it is not wise to abandon all drugs. Medication and other treatments can be useful in the appropriate setting and for appropriate illnesses, especially if you follow a risk versus benefit approach.

RISKY OR UNNECESSARY TESTS AND PROCEDURES

Trish was carving turkey in preparation for Thanksgiving dinner when her hand slipped. She knew the bright red stripe on the turkey breast was not gravy. Trish had cut her fingertip and, when the bleeding would not stop, went to an emergency room.

After a four-hour wait, the treating physician told her the laceration was small and would likely heal well. Trish had been nervous about the prospect of getting stitches. Based on what the doctor told her, she now believed she would leave the emergency room without stitches. Suddenly, Trish shivered when she heard the doctor's final pronouncement: "Might as well put in just two or three sutures."

While the doctor tied the last stitch, Trish could already feel sensation coming back to her numbed finger. She sat up, feet dangling over the side of the stretcher, her finger throbbing from the doctor's needle-work. She saw three stitches in a small cut on her swollen finger. Trish decided the experience was not as bad as she had imagined except for the brief pain while the doctor injected the numbing medication. The procedure, in fact, was far worse than Trish had thought. Since she asked no questions, she had no way of knowing that the suturing of her cut finger was largely unnecessary.

Trish fell victim to a potentially harmful procedure in that emergency room. Here are some of the possible reasons why the doctor chose to suture her finger cut, none of which were based on medical principles.

- "She came to the ER for treatment so she'll get a treatment" (whether she needs it or not). The adage, 'If you go to a barber, expect to get a haircut' holds true when seeking emergency or urgent care.
- "So she gets her money's worth after waiting so long."
- In an emergency room or office where they charge extra for each procedure, there is a few hundred dollars extra to be earned.
- In a teaching hospital, even a minor cut serves as good practice for a medical student or young doctor to learn suturing.

What is so bad about getting sutures? A wound will heal faster and with a smaller scar if stitches are necessary. Stitches, however, also pose risks such as infection, bleeding and needless pain, as well as added expense. More is not always better. Furthermore, inexperienced hands can cause deformity when a laceration is stitched improperly. Many other risky and useless procedures await your arrival in the emergency room and the reasons they are done would probably shock you.

When people seek help from an emergency room they expect the physician to take action. Many make comments such as: "Aren't you going to give me a prescription?" "Don't you think I should get an X ray?" "A blood test would give me peace of mind." These requests and demands by patients (as well as the prospect of future lawsuits) have sometimes persuaded or even coerced doctors into ordering tests or providing treatments that are not necessary.

In some ways, unnecessary high-tech procedures performed today are little different from healing rituals of primitive times. While there is greater scientific basis to modern therapies, avoidable death and dis-ability, as well as pain and suffering, are as tragic in a sterile ER treat-ment room as they were on the cold, bare ground in times past.

Long before the Hippocratic oath was written, trephining was a pop-ular "treatment" used for ailments such as headaches or convulsions.

During this procedure, the "healer" drilled holes into a patient's skull to release the demons believed to cause disease. These patients were awake! Sound barbaric? What about a procedure in which long needles and tubes are jabbed into an awake patient's groin and then threaded through the body into the heart?

If you do not recognize this gruesome procedure, it is an angiogram. The purpose of an angiogram is to locate blockages in the arteries that feed the heart with the hope of identifying any heart attacks waiting-to-happen. Once blocked arteries are discovered, three treatments are available and widely recommended. A patient can take heart medications that make it easier for the blood to flow through the blocked arteries and/or medicines to help prevent further blockages from forming. A riskier treatment called balloon angioplasty can be performed, in which a cardiologist mechanically unclogs cholesterol-filled arteries, like using a plumber's snake to unclog a toilet. Lastly, there is heart bypass surgery in which a surgeon sews in new blood channels around the blockages.

It may seem logical that the most tightly blocked artery is most likely to close off and cause a heart attack. But we now know an artery with *less* cholesterol plaque blockage can suddenly become totally blocked off first, leading to a heart attack. If a fresh blood clot forms, completely clogging that heart-feeding (coronary) artery, a heart attack is the result. An artery that is three-quarters blocked with cholesterol plaque will not always cause a heart attack before the half-clogged artery. This is unsettling news for the patient who underwent the risky balloon angioplasty to open up the artery that was three-quarters blocked. Furthermore, over one-third of "ballooned" arteries become blocked up again within several months. Even if performed by the most skilled cardiologist, about one in one hundred people who have an angioplasty procedure will die (this includes balloon dilatation; stenting, which is a wire mesh put in the artery to keep it open; and atherectomy, an artery cleaning procedure). As many as three in one hundred people will either have a heart attack or require emergency heart bypass surgery because of one of these procedures. You must ask yourself: Is the benefit worth the risk?

It must be questioned in each case whether an angioplasty procedure will improve a stable patient's outcome over treatment with medication alone. Furthermore, stable patients who undergo heart bypass surgery will not necessarily have a better long-term outcome than those only treated with medication. Why then is a heart angiogram (injecting dye into the heart-feeding arteries to check for blockages) done so freely if the ultimate treatments are not sufficiently beneficial for a large percentage of patients?

"New medicines and new methods of cure always work miracles—for a while," wrote the English physician William Heberden. Alarmingly, nearly fifty percent of angiograms done in this country are either unnecessary or could be postponed, according to a study published in the *Journal of the American Medical Association.*[4] Patients should open their eyes and understand that these wonder treatments and procedures have serious limitations and at times are no better than treating some patients with medications alone. A comparison study between the aggressive American approach to heart care and Canadian medicine's conservative heart care showed little difference in outcome.[5] The death rate and number of repeat heart attacks in the two countries were similar despite more angiograms, bypass surgeries and balloon angioplasties being performed in this country. Furthermore, another study[6] confirmed that heart attack patients who were brought to hospitals that offer high-tech heart treatments were more likely to undergo those procedures than people who were brought to hospitals without those resources. Having the latest technology available to you clearly can be a mixed blessing. On one hand, with these advanced technical procedures, the sickest patients' lives might be saved yet on the other hand, less serious heart attack patients might be subjected to needless risk or complications.

People often undergo unnecessary or avoidable procedures and tests in hospitals based on new treatment trends and established patterns of "proper" care. This algorithmic or "push button" approach to medicine is most evident in emergency rooms. Procedures are commonly performed without regard to an individual patient's need, tolerance or consequences. Doctors-in-training learn to manage medical problems by automatically ordering certain tests and performing specific actions, with little consideration of the potential risk for a particular patient.

TESTS AND PROCEDURES COMMONLY PERFORMED IN EMERGENCY ROOMS

The following tests are often necessary but at times, frequently avoidable, and sometimes done for reasons that are not medically sound.

Contrast or Dye Tests

Many iodine-containing contrast or dye tests are done from the emergency department, including CAT scan and intravenous pyelogram (IVP). Tests in which contrast dye is taken by mouth or inserted into the rectum are much safer than those in which the dye must be injected into a vein. The dye can cause complications such as kidney failure, particularly in diabetics and those who have preexisting kidney problems.

People who have asthma, hay fever, eczema, prior drug reactions or possibly a shellfish allergy may be at greater risk for developing an allergic reaction to contrast dye. Be sure "nonionic dye" is used in your test, because it is less likely to cause complications.

Gastric Lavage versus Endoscopy

A patient who vomits up a small amount of blood might be subjected to gastric lavage. Without any sedation, a plastic tube thicker than a pencil is inserted through the nose and down the back of the throat, finally reaching its destination in the stomach. Salt water is flushed into the stomach, then sucked out to see if the contents are clear and there is no sign of blood. This test sounds useful and it often does provide helpful information. Also, some patients must have a nasogastric (NG) tube inserted to help "rest" their stomach and through which nutritional supplements can be given. Many stable patients with bloody vomit, however, will also undergo endoscopy within a day or two. Endoscopy, the most accurate test, consists of a fiber-optic "scope" being inserted through the mouth and into the stomach (using sedation) to identify the cause of the bleeding. When this procedure is done early after a patient seeks care for bloody vomit—even those at low-risk for serious complications— endoscopy can help to reduce length of hospital stay, rates of recurrent bleeding, need for surgery, and death rate. Endoscopy can more accurately find the cause for bleeding than a nasogastric tube or X ray dye tests and, when found, the cause for bleeding can be treated during endoscopy.

Why subject a mildly ill patient with some bloody vomit to the nasogastric tube, too? Why not simply wait until the endoscopy can be performed in uncomplicated cases? Imagine having a long, flexible pencil shoved down your nose and throat when you are already nauseous and vomiting. Nasogastric tubes can also cause severe complications such as serious bleeding from the nose or a tear in the esophagus. Each case must be individualized and discussed with the patient in a risk versus benefit versus tolerance approach. Too often, patient tolerance and comfort is ignored and intolerable procedures are done automatically in the emergency room.

Clot-dissolving Drugs

Clot-dissolving medications such as tPA are routinely used in the first few hours after the symptoms of heart attack or stroke begin. Like using potent lye to unclog a pipe, clot-dissolving drugs help to open up an artery plugged by a fresh clot, the cause of most heart attacks and strokes. Unfortunately, however, these medications can cause bleeding anywhere in the body, including the brain.

At teaching hospitals, inexperienced doctors-in-training frequently give clot-dissolving drugs to heart attack patients. Quickly diagnosing a heart attack based on an electrocardiogram can be tricky even for experienced physicians. A young doctor can be fooled and administer this potentially dangerous drug to a person who is in fact not having a heart attack. A bleeding complication in this situation would be catastrophic as well as tragic, because it was totally unnecessary. Conversely, however, inexperienced doctors might miss the diagnosis of a heart attack, depriving some patients of the drug who, in fact, need this valuable treatment.

ABG Test

The arterial blood gases (ABG) test can be very painful. This procedure involves a deep needle stick into the wrist, arm or thigh to get a blood sample to measure pH, oxygen and carbon dioxide levels. This procedure can also be difficult to perform successfully and might require several painful attempts, particularly when done by doctors-in-training or rushed, overtaxed staff.

If you seek care at an emergency room for a complaint of shortness of breath, for instance, an ABG might be ordered even if your breathing problem improves quickly with simple treatment. The additional tests might be done to "document" on the chart that your lungs are working adequately should a problem arise after you have been sent home. Another reason the ABG might be needlessly performed is because of algorithmic medicine: "someone with breathing trouble must have a blood gas test done."

An oxygen monitor called a pulse oximeter is routinely available to painlessly measure oxygen levels in the blood. The pulse oximeter is a good alternative to an arterial blood gas test for less severe breathing problems. Consider this disturbing example of robotically performing a blood gas procedure without regard to patient tolerance and for dubious reason. In one case, a doctor-in-training insisted on performing an arterial blood gas test on an asthmatic patient. The patient protested, because his breathing nearly stopped the last time he was subjected to the same test. At that time, pain and anxiety from the needle sticks had made his asthma worse. The emergency room doctor in charge ultimately convinced the doctor-in-training to forego the ABG. That young doctor later admitted she was determined to do the test despite patient protests, because she feared being ridiculed at morning rounds for *not* having that particular test result. Patients are clearly not always the first consideration when tests or procedures are performed.

Back X Rays

A man lifts something heavy at work and wrenches his back. He feels agonizing muscle spasms in his lower back with any movement so he seeks
care at a nearby emergency room or urgent care facility. He feels reassured
when the doctor orders X rays of the lower back and tells him they were
okay. What the man does not know is that he was just exposed to about as
much radiation as if he had gotten one chest X ray daily for an entire year!
It is not just unnecessary radiation exposure that is a concern. A lower back
X ray on someone who lifts a heavy object or twists or turns wrong is
highly unlikely to show any useful information. Plain back X rays will not
show a slipped disc, pinched nerve or muscle or ligament damage. Plain
lower back X rays can be useful in older adults who are more likely to have
a collapsed vertebra or in people who fall from a ladder or sustain other serious back trauma. This man got an irrelevant test, was exposed to unnecessary radiation, and was given false reassurance that "his X ray was normal" which is meaningless for the type of injury he sustained.

Paronychia Overkill

What's that? Sounds terrible, but a paronychia is simply an infection, with
or without pus, of the skin adjacent to the fingernail (skin folds). The area
becomes red, swollen and exquisitely sensitive. Nail biting, hangnails, and
manicures contribute to this infection, which also tends to be more common in dishwashers, nurses and others with excessive hand exposure to
moisture. Finger-sucking in children also predisposes them to paronychia.
Sculptured fingernails have also been reported as a contributing factor.

Many doctors and other providers who treat this minor infection turn
a simple problem into a case of "treatments that are worse than the disease." Many doctors will treat paronychia in the following ways:

a) They might simply prescribe antibiotic pills and not drain the
pus to avoid a "time-consuming procedure." The infection is
not likely to clear any time soon until the pus is drained. Pain
will be prolonged, even if warm water soaks ultimately enable
the pus to drain out by itself.

b) The other side of the coin is the "overkill" approach in which an
anesthetic is injected on both sides of the base of the finger. This
can be quite painful if the novocaine is injected rapidly. A few
minutes later, the tip of the finger may or may not be completely
numb. Using a scalpel, an incision is then made over the inflamed
skin near the nail or a sharp instrument is jammed under the cuticle (skin fold) to lift that skin and allow the pus to drain. There is
usually a good deal of bleeding with either approach.

All that needs to be done to drain pus from a paronychia is to gently and painlessly scrape the bulging skin at the fold (near the cuticle) with a 25-gauge needle. Within three to five seconds the pus spurts out. Pressing the skin expresses any remaining pus. The pressing part is uncomfortable, but no other part of this twenty second procedure should be painful. Neither novocaine injections nor scalpel incisions are necessary to treat a paronychia. If the infection has not spread to the surrounding finger tissue, antibiotic pills are not required either. If there is no pus under the skin, then warm water soaks and antibiotic pills, as well as stopping the actions that led to the infection, are appropriate and sufficient treatment.

Joint Tap Risks

Emergency room doctors commonly drain fluid from joints using a fairly long needle, a procedure called arthrocentesis or "joint tap." The most important reason to perform this potentially painful and risky procedure is to diagnose a bacterial infection inside the joint (septic joint), which is a medical emergency. Sometimes doctors will want to drain a joint to try to diagnose the type of crystals causing pain such as gout. Another common reason to stick a long needle deep into a joint is to drain fluid or blood that has built up from an injury. The risks of this procedure are clear: pain if not adequately anesthetized, bleeding caused by the needle or a serious complication introducing infection into the joint. Most often, this procedure is elective, meaning it could be postponed until a more experienced doctor can do it (rheumatologist or orthopedist) or it can be avoided altogether if the swelling and pain improve quickly.

If a joint infection is a real possibility for a swollen and painful joint, a "joint tap" should be done immediately. Be certain the emergency or primary care doctor who performs this procedure has done many of these and is skilled at it. Better yet, ask for a rheumatologist or orthopedist to perform this risky procedure since they generally perform the most joint taps. Ultrasound guidance for needle placement can be helpful for difficult cases.

COSTLY TREATMENT DELAYS AND OUTRIGHT NEGLECT

Imagine being told, "We have an excellent treatment for your serious heart attack or stroke, but it's too late for you to benefit from it now." That's devastating news. The more time that passes after symptoms of a heart attack or stroke have begun, clot-dissolving treatment benefits drop considerably. For a heart attack, treatment should be initiated within the first one to two hours; for it to be effective, stroke treatment can only be given within three hours after symptoms come on. The longer the delay, the more risk individuals face relative to any benefit they might get from clot-dissolving treatments. Those who seek care at a hospital that offers angioplasty can benefit from the emergency opening of a clogged heart artery with a balloon and stent, a device placed in the artery to keep it open and unclogged. This treatment, in fact, is more successful than clot-dissolving drugs alone, but becomes less effective at saving lives when delays exceed one to two hours from the time of symptom onset.

Overcrowding as a major contributing factor to delays in getting care in the emergency room was discussed in Part One. Delays in getting prompt care for heart attack or stroke deserve special emphasis because their treatments are so time-dependent. The risks of clot-dissolving drugs and angioplasty may not be worth taking if you are treated beyond the time span in which they can offer the most benefit.

Treatment time delays can be divided into patient delays in seeking care and delays in getting clot-dissolving treatment once you arrive at an emergency room (door-to-needle time, as it is called). Experts recommend that *less* than **thirty minutes** should ensue from the time a patient arrives at the ER until a heart attack is diagnosed and the clot-dissolving medication is injected.

Stroke Treatment Delay

Millie was enjoying a lobster dinner at a charming restaurant. Her daughter had just graduated magna cum laude from a prestigious university and Millie glowed with pride. Millie's daughter, Sondra, was telling a joke and everyone at the table listened with anticipation. Halfway through the story, Sondra noticed butter sauce seeping out from the right corner of her mother's mouth. She continued toward the punch line, intermittently glancing at her mother. Soon, the joke completed, laughter erupted at the table. Another glance her mother's way, however, and Sondra knew something was wrong. Only the left corner of Millie's mouth curved upward with her smile. The right side of Millie's mouth drooped downward and saliva dribbled out.

"Are you alright, Mother?" Sondra asked nervously.

"Yes," Millie mumbled, waving her hand.

Millie sounded drunk, but she never drank alcohol. Millie reassured her daughter that she was fine, but a few minutes later she reached over for a napkin and fell off her chair, crashing down onto the wooden floor.

Sondra jumped up and pleaded for someone to call for an ambulance. She called out her mother's name and Millie's eyes opened. Sondra realized her mother's right arm and leg remained still.

Once inside the emergency room, a busy nurse stared with narrowed eyes at the ambulance technician who wheeled Millie in. "Fourth patient in an hour. Can't you go to St. Joe's ER next time?" the nurse asked.

"Just a stroke patient," the technician replied.

"Oh, good. What's her pressure?"

"Sky high—two-twenty over one-thirty."

"Room six down the hall," the nurse said.

That nurse did not return to check Millie's blood pressure for fifteen minutes. The doctor on duty was treating another patient and was told about Millie thirty minutes after her arrival. He ordered blood pressure-lowering medication that was given nearly forty minutes after she arrived. Meanwhile, Millie's arm and leg became heavier and more immobile. Nobody could know if some of her deterioration might have been prevented with faster action in the emergency room.

Was it Millie's fate to be paralyzed from her stroke? Could *immediate* blood pressure treatment have minimized her disability? Delays in treating skyrocketing blood pressure can amount to microscopic cellular murder as damaged brain cells shrivel and self-destruct. Patients who suffer a stroke are frequently neglected in the emergency room as doctors and nurses expend their efforts on "more treatable" illnesses. While it is true that few patients prove to be eligible for treatment to stop a stroke, the National Stroke Association guidelines emphasize that more rapidly stopping brain injury increases chances for recovery.

Clot-dissolving treatment is now available for most strokes if given within three hours after symptoms begin. Some causes for delay at the hospital include the doctor recognizing the diagnosis of stroke and getting a CAT scan done. At community or smaller hospitals, this can involve calling CAT scan technicians into the hospitals from their homes during late-night hours.

A CAT scan or MRI of the brain must first be performed to distinguish which of two types of stroke the patient is experiencing: a bleed into the brain or a blood clot blocking nourishment to brain cells. These two forms of stroke are treated differently, but with both types earlier action can mean fewer cells will die. Strokes caused by a blood clot can now be treated with clot-dissolving medication. If a brain bleed causes a stroke, blood pressure must be carefully and quickly lowered if it is

exceedingly high. By the time Millie received proper medication to nor-
malize her blood pressure, her arm and leg were nearly paralyzed. Could
permanent paralysis have been avoided with earlier action? Possibly.
What can be said with certainty, is that Millie should not have had to
wait forty minutes before action was taken to treat her.

Heart Attacks: "Time is Muscle"

In an ER, a forty-eight-year-old man with trouble breathing is hooked
up to a heart monitor and oxygen. He is changed into a hospital gown
and an intravenous line is placed in his forearm. The nurses are very
busy so they call the electrocardiogram technician to perform the EKG.
By the time she arrives and does the EKG, fifty minutes have elapsed
since the man arrived. The technician must rush back to the intensive
care unit because they keep paging her so she rests the EKG down on
the nurse's station counter and hurries upstairs. Another thirty minutes
pass before the busy, lone emergency doctor evaluates the patient,
locates the electrocardiogram, diagnoses a heart attack and initiates
clot-dissolving treatment.

Such frivolous delays are inexcusable and have serious consequences. After all, "Time is muscle." Many studies confirm that both
clot-dissolving treatment and balloon angioplasty are far more effective
in saving lives when treatment is provided within **one to two hours** of
symptom onset. While patients themselves frequently delay seeking
help, many ER internal system factors can contribute to emergency
department delays in commencing treatment. In fact, some studies
found that more than a thirty-minute delay can increase chances for
death by nearly ten percent, while delays greater than ninety minutes
can increase chances for death by twenty-seven percent!

Less typical symptoms of heart attack can cause confusion in diagnosis and treatment delays, leading to patients receiving fewer appropriate treatments. Smaller hospitals without heart catheterization labs have
been found to generally increase risk for treatment delay. Some studies
have found advanced age, being female and having either diabetes or
heart failure to be associated with greater ER treatment delays for heart
attack. Subtle or hard to read electrocardiogram abnormalities and treatment by inexperienced doctors can also lead to greater delays.

In the previous example, the forty-eight-year-old heart attack victim came for help immediately, but slow and inefficient work in the ER
cost him his best chance for survival and recovery.

Neglect is an everyday occurrence in emergency rooms resulting in
harm the consequences of which cannot be measured. Consider these

commonplace examples of neglect that can happen in any busy ER, as reported by Drs. Derlet and Richard in their *Annals of Emergency Medicine* article titled, "Overcrowding in the Nation's Emergency Departments: Complex Causes and Disturbing Effects."[7]

A woman goes unevaluated for several hours as she lies on a stretcher in an emergency room. Her temperature was not taken. In fact, she suffered from hyperthermia, a potentially fatal overheated state of the body.

A patient sat in a hallway for nearly eight hours without a thorough evaluation during a busy, overcrowded period in an ER. Ultimately, he was diagnosed with a potentially fatal blood clot in the brain.

While it may be understandable when an emergency room and its staff is overtaxed, such neglect is disturbing, dangerous and may be deadly. However, even if not fatal, the pain and injury caused by the following common lapses in emergency room care are unacceptable and avoidable.

Hemorrhages Out of Control

The ambulance crew wheels a woman into a community hospital emergency room at 2:00 A.M. The woman is hemorrhaging from a bleeding stomach ulcer. She just vomited red blood and has had bloody diarrhea. Her breathing status: moderate distress with a breathing rate twice normal. Blood pressure: eighty systolic—life threatening. The emergency doctor and nurse start two large intravenous lines while blood for transfusion is ordered from the blood bank. Salt-rich fluids pour into the woman's depleted veins and her blood pressure creeps higher. Suddenly, a page on the overhead speaker: "Code blue CCU." The emergency room doctor must stop treatment for this seriously ill woman and rush upstairs to treat a patient in the Coronary Care Unit. Upstairs, the patient's heart had just stopped. Many community hospitals have a policy in which the emergency room doctor must immediately go onto the hospital floors to treat critically ill hospital patients when no other doctors are available. While the ER doctor was upstairs, the woman with the bleeding ulcer in the emergency room developed complications. Her condition deteriorated and she died. The patient upstairs had little chance of being saved, but the woman with a bleeding ulcer might have lived had she received the doctor's undivided attention.

Dangerous Humiliation

An elderly woman falls on ice and breaks her hip. While she waits in the emergency room, she calls for twenty minutes for a bedpan, but is ignored by busy staff. Unable to wait any longer, she soils herself and must sit in her feces for thirty minutes more before a nurse's aid cleans her. Not only is this neglect humiliating, it can also lead to bedsores and other serious complications.

Pain Prolonged

A man with side pain is told to sit out in the waiting room. He does not utter a word despite his agonizing pain. After a three-hour wait, the doctor examines him and suspects a kidney stone. The stoic man waits an additional twenty minutes before the nurse gives him a shot of pain medication. The man waited nearly four hours for assistance even though kidney stone pain is considered to be one of the worst types of pain an individual can experience.

The emergency room proved to be a two-edged sword for Bob, Trish and Millie and it can happen to you, too. Each time you pass through those metal emergency room doors, like walking through the jungle, anything can happen. Your life might be saved—or scarred and changed forever. Bob fell victim to a treatment that proved to be worse than the disease. Trish was subjected to one of many unnecessary procedures on the "ER procedure menu." And Millie's life might have been forever changed by neglect, which is, unfortunately, a common treatment modality in our nation's overwhelmed emergency departments.

HOW DO YOU SIDESTEP HARM?

All doctors take the oath to "first do no harm," but you must help them to uphold it. As a healthcare consumer, each person must always play the role of skeptic or devil's advocate when being diagnosed or treated for a medical problem, especially when receiving emergency care. With the help of your treating doctor, discuss your situation thoroughly and do a risk-benefit analysis to determine if the potential gains of any intervention justify possible risks.

Remember to always expect the unexpected with regard to tests, treatments and procedures. A recent study published in the February 2001 issue of the *New England Journal of Medicine* teaches this lesson quite clearly.[8] The study showed that many mental functions such as concentration and memory declined significantly in nearly half of patients who underwent coronary artery bypass surgery. This shocking finding comes after decades of "perfecting" this serious surgery to the point of making it routine. Who would have guessed that those who undergo this heart surgery might come out of it with a new and improved heart, but perhaps a declining mind?

A risk-benefit analysis considers potential gains and their likelihood versus the probability of complications such as death or disability. An excellent example of a risk-benefit analysis is a woman deciding to take hormone replacement therapy. Possible benefits include reducing chances for osteoporosis, lessening the intensity and duration of hot flashes and perhaps helping reduce heart disease risk. Risks of hormone replacement therapy include increased chances for cancer of the uterus and breast and side effects such as fluid retention and headaches. Each woman must weigh the pros and cons to decide what is best in her individual situation.

One giant step toward the goal of preventing harm is to take an active role in your own or a loved one's medical care. Ask questions. Insist on being informed. No matter how busy, it is a doctor's obligation to satisfactorily explain to a patient the pros and cons of a test or treatment that the doctor has recommended. Do not allow the doctor to skimp on or rush through this crucial responsibility. *Your* life and health are at stake.

IMPORTANT QUESTIONS TO ASK
ABOUT COMMON TESTS AND PROCEDURES

Before you agree to a test, procedure or treatment get common sense answers to these questions:

- *What is the goal of the test or treatment and how likely is it to succeed?*
  For example, it is not advisable to take an antibiotic if the doctor is confident that you suffer from a viral infection which is unaffected by antibiotics. As another example, think hard before agreeing to risky clot-dissolving treatment for a **mild** heart attack if it is being given more than six hours after symptoms began. The benefits may be minimal when getting the treatment so late.

- *Will that test or procedure provide information that will change the treatment plan?*
  Why X-ray a stubbed toe to check for a broken bone if the treatment is to tape the toe whether it is bruised or broken? Remember the case of the man with the wrenched back who was given an irrelevant lower back X ray and be sure that the test or procedure being proposed for you is appropriate for your type of injury or illness.

- *What are the most common and worst risks of the test or treatment?*
  If you take an antibiotic, for instance, the most common risk might be stomach upset while the worst risk, although uncommon, is a deadly anaphylactic allergic reaction. While the clot dissolving drug tPA can stop a heart attack in its tracks, in some cases it can

also cause a deadly brain bleed. Don't be afraid to know the good and the bad about a test or treatment and do your risk-benefit analysis.

- *Are there safer alternatives?*
A sonogram of the kidneys can sometimes provide enough information to check for a kidney problem rather than a CAT scan with contrast dye. The CAT scan exposes patients to radiation and the potential risks of intravenous contrast dye such as kidney failure or a bad allergic reaction. Why take a potent medication when a simple, safer treatment may suffice? If you don't ask about alternatives, however, they may not be offered or suggested.

- *Are there safe and simple measures to try first?*
For some illnesses, dietary modifications, exercise, lifestyle changes, weight loss and other basic measures should always be considered first. You would be foolhardy to take long-term medication to treat high blood pressure with its many possible side effects before trying diet and weight-loss measures.

- *What are the risks of a watch and wait approach?*
If an illness is likely to heal on its own, you should not undergo risky tests or allow avoidable treatments. For instance, there is no need to take antibiotic pills for a minor skin infection that is likely to heal by cleaning it with soap and water. A diabetic, who is susceptible to serious infection, on the other hand, may be better off taking the antibiotic pills. Once again, do your risk-benefit analysis of the situation.

INFORMED CONSENT

Your active participation in deciding whether a test, procedure or treatment will be performed or prescribed, and the physician's explanation of risks, benefits, alternatives and accepted medical knowledge about that test or treatment all constitute informed consent. Informed consent is based on the legal principle that every competent adult has the right to choose what is done with his or her own body. A person can consent to or refuse any medical intervention after a healthcare professional explains relevant information. Patients have a right to expect a reasonable amount of time for an explanation, not a pressured one-minute conversation. A doctor should always allow a patient to ask questions and should respond patiently and thoroughly, even though this can sometimes be difficult in a hectic, pressured ER setting. Remember, however, that it is your health and perhaps your life at stake, so ask questions.

What Information is Relevant?

- The general nature of the test, treatment or procedure
- Anticipated benefits and chances for success
- Most serious and most common risks
- Reasonable alternatives to that intervention and their risks/benefits
- Pros and cons of doing nothing

How much information is enough? Every locale, be it state, county or court jurisdiction, abides by one of two standards: the Professional Standard or the Lay Standard. Based on the Professional Standard, a healthcare provider must disclose the type and amount of information that other similar physicians would disclose. The Lay (or Material Risk) Standard dictates that the type and amount of information disclosed be adequate for any reasonable person in that patient's shoes. Would any person want or expect certain information before deciding on that intervention? With the Lay Standard, the focus is centered on the patient.

Informed consent can only be valid if the person agreeing to a test or treatment is a competent adult who is not *impaired* by drugs or disease. Adequate information must be disclosed and the patient or the patients' surrogate, if the patient is not competent or is impaired to such an extent that comprehension is impossible, must understand the explanation. Interpreters, hearing aids, reading materials, videos and Internet information resources can and should be used to achieve the goal of patient comprehension. Consent must also be voluntary. Some ethicists argue that untreated severe pain can be a form of medical coercion since the patient might undergo the procedure only because of the promise of pain relief from the treatment.

There are, of course, exceptions to these requirements. Life or limb-threatening emergency can override the need for informed consent and so can mental incompetence in a patient who has no surrogate to make decisions on his or her behalf.

Interesting Points to Bear in Mind Relevant to Informed Consent:

- The manner in which a doctor frames or describes risks can have a major influence on a patient's decision. That is why a patient should assume the role of skeptic and take the vantage point of a worst possible case scenario. For instance, if a doctor told you angioplasty to unclog a heart-feeding artery is ninety-nine percent safe, you would feel reassured. What if the doctor said that one in every one hundred people who undergo angioplasty will die, meaning thousands of people among the hundreds of thousands who undergo the procedure annually. Suddenly, the procedure doesn't sound so innocuous any more, does it?

- In one study of patients suffering from active heart problems, the data showed that only a minority of patients remembered the risks of a particular treatment, while a large majority remembered the benefits.[9] Wishful thinking or selective memory will not help when you are deciding whether or not to undergo a risky treatment. A trusted relative or friend serving as patient advocate comes in handy at these times for discussing and reviewing options, as well as reminding the patient of information that may have been overlooked or forgotten.
- In those patients who were undergoing an elective heart procedure like angioplasty, one study found the majority of patients had unrealistic expectations about long-term benefits and less than half of the patients were able to recall even one risk!

It is within your rights as patient to refuse a test or treatment offered to you by a physician. "I'm sorry, but I'll pass on that test for now" will not offend a competent, confident and compassionate doctor.

CAREFULLY CONSIDER ANY TREATMENTS

A few suggestions to avoid the all too common dilemma of seeking care for one illness and ending up with an even worse medical problem:

1. After you have asked the appropriate questions discussed earlier, press the doctor for some hard facts about the chances for success, death or disability. For instance, surgery for many lower back problems does not fully eliminate the pain. How much better are you likely to get to justify the risk?
2. Never make a decision about a risky procedure before consulting trusted relatives and your family doctor and without getting a second (and perhaps third) opinion from a specialist or other trusted professional.
3. Be sure to take the skeptic or devil's advocate view so you clearly see the risks involved.
4. Ask about all treatment options. Researchers have recently found that clot-dissolving treatment used in heart attack sufferers over age seventy-five caused twice as many deaths as those who did not get that treatment. Those who are over age seventy-five might be better off getting emergency angioplasty to unclog an artery during a heart attack, a treatment causing far fewer brain bleeds and strokes.

A treatment that works for "most people" is not necessarily best for you.

5. The best defense is a strong offense. Ask questions. If this is not a life or death emergency situation and time permits, do medical research on the World Wide Web to get relevant information and names of medical experts for special procedures.

6. Be suspicious of a doctor who does not ask for your input in making decisions about your care. Do not settle for fluffy answers like, "You have nothing to worry about, it's very safe."

SAY 'NO' TO RISKY AND UNNECESSARY TESTS OR TREATMENTS

Politely refuse "just-in-case" tests or treatments that might do more harm than good. Will a test result actually change the treatment plan? If not, pass. It is your right to refuse. Another important consideration is whether you can tolerate such a test or treatment based on your pain tolerance and degree of illness. Again, if your situation and time permits, get opinions from trusted relatives, friends and other medical professionals as to whether a test or treatment is worth the risk. Allow less serious ailments some time (one to three days) to improve before seeking aggressive treatment.

AVOID DELAYS AND NEGLECT

Asking questions or refusing a test or treatment are fairly simple to do, but solutions are limited for treatment delays and neglect in the ER. The overcrowding and understaffing problems in our nation's emergency departments will not be solved any time soon.

When you suddenly become ill or sustain an injury, first inform your family doctor that you are going to the emergency room. If you already have a relationship with a quality physician, he or she might meet and examine you in the emergency room, bypassing the wait for the emergency room doctor. Be sure you go to or are taken to a hospital in which your family physician has privileges. Alternatively, your doctor might suggest seeing you in the office for less serious problems, an advantage of an ongoing and trusting relationship with your family doctor.

Once you have decided to go to the emergency room it is prudent to go with a friend or relative, not alone. Your companion can serve as your advocate, telling a nurse or doctor if you are still in pain or need a urinal. A companion can send out a gentle reminder to the ER staff that your blood pressure has not been rechecked in quite a while even though the original plan was to recheck it within one hour. The advocate must be polite, not rude or challenging, or he or she will make enemies quickly. The advocate must prioritize those issues worth pursuing. Friends and family who constantly make demands on already overburdened emergency workers will alienate themselves and the patient. Polite requests phrased in this manner, "When you get a chance, my mother is still in pain," go a long way with overtaxed ER personnel. The staff might become angry and hostile and make you wait longer for irate comments like "My mother is being neglected here and she's still in pain!" Remember, when a new, seriously ill patient arrives in the emergency department, you become old news. You or your advocate must politely seek out the attention you deserve.

Some additional tips to sidestep ER delays:

- When you arrive at an emergency room and find it overcrowded with people practically hanging from the rafters, consider (if you physically can) trying a nearby community hospital emergency room instead. Call ahead and ask if they, too, are experiencing total chaos. They won't give details but might make comments such as: "It's crazy here, too." or "Things aren't too bad."
- For less serious, walk-in problems, if you decide to seek emergency care, first consider carefully the day of the week and time of day. Mondays are always busy in emergency rooms as well as medical offices, as a rule. Friday and Saturday nights tend to get very busy in ERs. Studies have shown that less than ten percent of ER patients are seen between 4:00 to 8:00 A.M. But remember: you might be awakening a sleeping doctor who may be groggy and not alert.
- Try to get your doctor to meet you at the emergency room (if he or she feels you are better off going there rather than the office). Your family doctor can streamline your care in the ER. Perhaps your doctor will be willing to admit you, if necessary, directly into the hospital if beds are available.

How To Avoid ER Treatment Delays For Chest Pain Or Heart Attacks

The single best way to prevent treatment delay for chest pain or possible heart attack is to learn the common and uncommon symptoms of a heart attack and to seek help immediately. If you have a cardiologist or internist, you or a relative should call your doctor to alert him or her to your problem. Hopefully, the doctor will meet you in the ER, particularly if you have a history of serious heart problems. Some additional tips:

- Call 911 and request an ambulance. Do not go to the hospital by car and walk into the ER, if possible. You will be seen faster by doctors when you bypass the waiting room and desk clerk sign-in (the clerk will come to you or a family member while you are being treated or evaluated) and, in the ambulance, treatment can be initiated en route.
- The goal of heart attack care is to provide definitive treatment within thirty minutes after a patient arrives in the emergency room. A family member or friend should ask about an electrocardiogram (EKG), if one has not been done within ten minutes after arrival at the emergency department. Be certain the nurse or EKG technician hands the EKG paper to the doctor! It is not unusual for an EKG to sit in a chart or on a countertop for many precious minutes until the doctor gets to it or realizes it has been completed.
- Some rural communities have considered allowing paramedics to administer clot-dissolving medication during the long trip to the hospital. This can be a great timesaver for obvious heart attacks, but this process also increases the risks of mistaken judgment by less trained and inexperienced professionals.
- Consider using a hospital emergency room in your area that offers a chest pain evaluation unit. Especially if you are aware that you have heart problems, it makes sense to learn which hospital(s) nearby maintains this type of diagnostic unit.

Chest Pain Evaluation Units

A growing number of emergency departments are setting up chest pain units to improve care for heart patients. Most of these units remain closely linked to the main emergency room and do not necessarily have a completely separate and specially trained staff.

The purpose of these units is to avoid mistakenly discharging patients who might have a heart problem. Heart attacks and angina are frequently *not* obvious or clear cut. Another goal of Chest Pain Evaluation Units is to avoid admitting someone into the hospital if they are unlikely to have a true heart problem. Those who clearly do have a heart attack or angina benefit by receiving prompt and appropriate treatment.

Chest pain units have protocols set up for serial blood tests and EKGs, physical examinations over time, heart monitoring, and needed medications. After a six to twelve hour period of observation, if any doubt remains as to whether a patient has a heart problem, specialized tests that are variations of a stress test will be performed before sending a patient home (or keeping that person in the hospital). While these stress tests are not perfect, they can provide additional useful information.

As they are relatively new, it is not yet clear if chest pain units actually achieve their patient care goals, but they are surely a step in the right direction. However, the name "chest pain unit" is problematic. Since up to one-third of heart attacks do *not* involve chest pain, the title can be misleading to patients and others who will be under the mistaken impression that without chest pain, there can be no heart attack. Also, many heart attack sufferers do not consider their chest symptoms to be an actual "pain."

Avoiding ER Treatment Delays For Stroke

Time delays for stroke can have tragic as well as permanent consequences. Lackadaisical or haphazard emergency treatment of patients with stroke is no longer acceptable. A stroke victim's family member or friend acting as patient advocate will be essential in obtaining prompt treatment in a busy ER.

The National Stroke Association has issued new guidelines on stroke treatment. Both doctors and patients are urged to learn and take seriously the signs and symptoms of a stroke. Symptoms include weakness or numbness in a limb, slurred speech, headache and visual disturbances. A stroke should be considered a "brain attack" and must be treated as aggressively as a heart attack. Certain strokes can now be treated with clot-dissolving drugs if diagnosed within three hours of onset of symptoms. Call 911 if you suffer symptoms that might be a stroke. Do not allow someone to drive you unless the wait for an ambulance will be longer than the time it takes to drive to an ER.

As a potential ER patient, the most valuable advice you can glean from this section of the book is to remember to ask pertinent questions about your care and treatment. Stay alert or be sure to have someone with you acting as your advocate. Participate in your own or a loved one's care. Insist on thorough explanations of what your diagnosis is, tests or treatments that are available and major risks involved. This approach will help protect you in the often intimidating, jungle-like atmosphere of the emergency room.

USEFUL WEB SITES

http://www.yoursurgery.com
   (Surgical procedures explained by surgeons through diagrams, photos and animation.)

http://health.discovery.com/diseasesandcond/encyclopedia medical_tests_encyclopedia.html
(This site provides information on a broad range of medical tests including how to prepare for them, what to expect and what the results mean.)

http://www.sav-ondrugs.com
(An online drugstore that offers over-the-counter and prescription medication as well as general merchandise.)

http://www.adam.com
(This site provides health information on a wide range of diseases, tests, procedures, etc., using illustrations, 3-D models and other methods.)

http://drkoop.com/conditions/ency
(This medical enyclopedia page is part of the consumer health information site started by former Surgeon General C. Everett Koop.)

http://www.americanheart.org/statistics
(This site provides the American Heart Association's statistical updates on heart and stroke hospitalizations, costs and deaths.)

http://www.stroke.org
(This is the Web site of the National Stroke Association, a group dedicated to fighting strokes and helping those at risk, suffering or recovering from this condition.)

http://www.strokecenter.org
(Sponsored by the Washington University Medical Center, this site offers information for patients, their families and health professionals.)

http://www.nhlbi.nih.gov
(The National Heart, Lung and Blood Institute's Web site provides information for patients and doctors.)

http://www.cdc.gov
(This is the Centers for Disease Control and Prevention's Web site.)

DANGER #2
MEDICAL ERRORS, ADVERSE EVENTS
AND OTHER NOXIOUS PROBLEMS

Doctors kill as many as 98,000 hospitalized people every year, according to a 1999 report on patient harm published by the respected Institute of Medicine (IOM). Some medical organizations and experts have questioned the science behind the IOM report, but its basic premise is indisputable: Medical errors cause permanent disability, avoidable suffering and many deaths in American hospitals. Where does the cycle of patient harm begin? Behind those metal doors, inside the emergency room.

In truth, the number of medical miscues (known as adverse events) is probably much greater. Adverse events that are identifiable are merely the tip of the medical error iceberg. For example, standard hospital self-reporting systems miss approximately ninety-five percent of medication mistakes![10] Imagine how many treatment errors go unnoticed when nobody knows exactly what is wrong with a seriously ill patient. If the wrong treatment is given for an uncertain illness, both healthcare workers and family might assume the patient died from serious illness and not failure to get proper treatment. The man in heart failure who improperly gets too much intravenous fluids and stops breathing—he died from a weak heart, not carelessness. An agitated elderly patient gets restrained and sedated. It was actually an overlooked blood infection that caused her agitation and, ultimately, her death. All her family will ever know is that she died of a severe infection and old age.

It is not just the fatal errors that remain hushed and hidden and unnoticed. No statistics are tallied on avoidable patient suffering and disability. A young woman develops lower abdominal pain and is subjected to several pelvic examinations by a student, an intern and more experienced doctors during her emergency room visit. The tears this woman shed are cried in vain. Her vaginal soreness and humiliation are not recorded as an adverse event. When clot-dissolving treatment is delayed for a stroke or heart attack patient, more viable cells shrivel and die. Residual disability might have been avoided with faster treatment. But who will ever know? These are the risks you take when you enter this often chaotic, clamorous environment that may be overtaxed and staffed by many inexperienced or inadequately trained healthcare providers who are tired and overworked.

To receive quality emergency medical care, a person cannot simply plop onto the stretcher and wait for excellent medical care to happen. It might not. Medical errors are plentiful even at the most prestigious hospitals. Discord and overcrowding, plus inexperienced or inadequately trained workers make the emergency department fertile ground for damaging or even lethal mistakes. The following statistics might scare you right out of any hospital or emergency room, but if you have made yourself knowledgeable about the system, there is no need to bolt. These frightening facts clearly illustrate why every patient must stay informed, remain alert or, if that is impossible, have someone there to serve as an advocate and actively participate in testing and treatment decisions to help medical professionals avoid errors and provide quality emergency or hospital care. An aware patient can "keep 'em on their toes!"

- About 7000 people die every year because of medication errors including prescribing and dispensing the wrong drugs, according to the recent Institute of Medicine report on medical errors.
- For every one hundred people suffering a heart attack, between two and eight people will be sent home from the emergency room with the wrong diagnosis.[11]
- According to the Harvard Medical Practice Study I (which studied known adverse events in tens of thousands of people), medical errors occurred in about four of every one hundred hospitalized patients. Nearly fourteen percent of these errors led to death! About three percent of these errors led to permanent disability. Half of these bad treatment outcomes were preventable, according to the study.
- The Harvard Medical Practice Study II found that a high rate of emergency department adverse events were due to misdiagnosis.
- The elderly suffer more preventable adverse events than younger patients, according to research published in the *British Medical Journal*. Older patients had a higher incidence of preventable adverse events from medical procedures (such as heart catheterization and bronchoscopy), adverse drug events and preventable falls.[12]
- During the initial emergency room evaluation, an electrocardiogram diagnoses a heart attack in only one half of patients who later prove to have a heart attack. Tests, too, are inherently fallible.

These are frightening facts, but do not despair. Use the following basic and common sense precautions to increase your chances for error-free, quality care in the ER.

DO NOT ALLOW YOURSELF TO BECOME A STATISTIC

Don't be a passive, "Whatever you say, Doc" type of patient. Ask questions and expect explanations: it will keep medical professionals on the ball. If you are the shy type, cannot question authority or if you are just too ill, then bring along a friend or relative who will serve as your patient advocate. Follow these common sense tips and you are well on your way to avoiding detrimental emergency care and treatment.

PLAN AHEAD TO MAKE KEY ER DECISIONS

Avoid the emergency room whenever possible. The emergency room is a dynamic, often tense environment with patients moving from one place or test to another and ER workers going from one patient to another. Staff and patients have usually never met before so any degree of familiarity is lacking. What's more, decisions are made in an eye-blink with few, if any, checks and balances in the emergency room setting. Even medications are usually prepared and administered by ER staff without benefit of double-checking for proper medication and dose by pharmacy staff. The rushed, chaotic nature of the ER is a setup for miscommunications, misdiagnoses and mistakes. A few tips:

- Stick to one hospital and/or doctor whenever possible (except for trauma, pediatric and invasive heart care). With too many cooks in your healthcare kitchen, your recipe for health might get ruined. Fragmented care leads to errors when doctors and nurses do not know you and do not have access to all your medical records.
- Use a high volume hospital for high-tech procedures such as angioplasty or heart catheterization. When the most experienced hands perform procedures, outcomes are generally better. For instance, eight operations were found in a study to have a significantly higher risk of preventable adverse events: artery bypass graft of legs, repair of aortic aneurysm in the abdomen, removal of large intestine, heart bypass or valve surgery, transurethral resection of prostate (TURP) or bladder tumor surgery, gallbladder removal, hysterectomy (uterus removal) and appendectomy.[13] The most experienced surgeon should perform pediatric surgery at a well-equipped hospital. Ask your surgeon if he or she or less experienced doctors-in-training will actually perform the operation.
- Adopt a "say-no-to-tests" attitude. Agree to tests only if your doctor gives you compelling, common sense reasons why you should have it done. Use the same approach for risky treatments as well. Second opinions are recommended before you agree to undergo a

major operation or invasive procedure for an illness that is not immediately life threatening.

- Remember that doing nothing can sometimes be the best medicine. Allow time for self-healing with less serious ailments.
- If you are over age forty or have any heart problems or recurrent chest pains, carry in your purse or wallet a miniaturized and laminated copy of your baseline electrocardiogram. Comparing a new electrocardiogram with an old one can increase accuracy in diagnosing heart problems.
- Have emergency staff check with your family doctor for more medical history when you have a troubling symptom or before undergoing risky tests or treatments.

AVOID MISDIAGNOSIS:
A COMMON CAUSE OF ADVERSE EVENTS

In the helter-skelter world of emergency rooms and urgent care offices, a patient can do all the right things and still get burned. A woman with severe indigestion promptly seeks medical care. She knows something is not right. The emergency care doctor gets basic blood tests and orders a sonogram to check for gallstones. There are none. The blood tests are fine. She still feels quite ill and seems to be getting worse, not better. The doctor comes to her bedside and says, "Good news, the tests were all normal so you can go home now. Your pain should improve over the next few days with antacids and Tylenol and follow up with your family doctor."

"But I'm feeling worse," the lady says.

"Sometimes you get worse before getting better," the doctor explains.

"But I don't think this is indigestion. I've had that before and this seems different," the woman replies.

"Give it a few days and call your family MD," the doctor says reassuringly.

Normal test results do not mean a thing for a patient who is in pain and deteriorating. Of course the woman had normal test results that showed no problems with her stomach—she actually had a heart problem, not a stomach disorder. The wrong tests were ordered, thus, the diagnosis was plainly incorrect.

Never assume medical workers are always correct when they tell you something that defies common sense. Do not hesitate to get a second opinion when you are or a loved one is seriously ill or getting *worse* after an evaluation and simple treatment. Emergency room or urgent care providers often say that since nothing turned up on the tests, it must be something that should get better at home in a few days. A patient must insist that he or she feels *worse* or just as bad as before and firmly request a specialist or more experienced doctor who can determine the nature and extent of the illness. Needless to say, this should be done only for potentially serious illness, not a lingering cold or cough. Remember, tests are imperfect! Serious illness does manifest itself in different people in unusual ways that defy textbook descriptions. It is not rare for high-tech tests (or those who interpret them) to miss a serious problem. Moreover, if a person seeks care before a serious illness has "blossomed" into overt symptoms, it can easily mislead even a doctor with fine clinical judgment. It is also not uncommon for doctors to simply be off the mark if they jump to a conclusion too early or if they are not experienced enough to recognize unusual presentations of serious illness.

What can you do if a doctor wants to send you home from the emergency room or hospital, but you feel worse and are concerned (with good reason) that it might be serious? The first step is to have the ER doctor call your family doctor to discuss your case. At that time, you can voice your concerns to your family doctor. If that does not work, ask your family doctor to come to the ER to evaluate you or have the emergency care doctor call in a specialist for another opinion.

Lastly, you can speak with the hospital's **Patient Advocate or Patient Representative**. This person serves as a voice of reason and a link between you and everyone else in the hospital including medical staff and administrators. The Patient Representative can perhaps help to arrange a reasonable compromise that benefits everyone, such as a night of hospital observation and reevaluation to see if you improve or continue to feel worse.

BE ALERT TO MEDICATION ERRORS

Politely refuse medications and prescriptions unless the doctor provides logical and compelling reasons why you should take the drug. As a rule, if you must take medication, request safer and cheaper alternatives. Here are a few more helpful hints:

- Computerized and E-mail prescriptions should help to eliminate many medication errors in the future. Until that time, if a doctor hands you a necessary prescription with half the words looking like hieroglyphics, politely ask the doctor to rewrite it more legibly. The pharmacist could misread that prescription.

- Know all medications that you take. Carry a list in your wallet. Look at the pictures inside the *Physicians Desk Reference* to learn what the drug looks like.
- Remember to mention to the doctor all over-the-counter medications, herbals or health supplements you have been taking. These can cause serious side effects or interact with other medications.
- Never take any medication while in the emergency room or hospital unless you know what it is, the dosage, what it is for and *who* ordered it.
- If anyone gives you a medication, mention your drug allergies and those medications you cannot tolerate due to side effects. Be sure your drug allergies are updated in your chart.
- Ask your doctor if any other drugs have strikingly similar names to your medication. This might help to avoid a prescribing error down the road.
- Avoid newfangled medications when old reliable drugs can do the job. Several new drugs have been found to cause serious side effects shortly after they were approved by the FDA for common use.
- If you suffer from liver or kidney disease, tell your doctor or nurse. Medication dosage might need to be adjusted.
- When taking any new medication report to your doctor any strange feelings or ailments you experience. It might be a side effect which could prove to be harmful.
- If you agree to take a medication, use it for the shortest length of time *that will still be effective*. This might help to avoid a side effect, allergic reaction or antibiotic resistance. There is no clear scientific basis to treat common infections such as sinusitis or middle ear infection for ten days or longer, for instance. Also, numerous studies have found that short course appropriate antibiotics for certain types of infections (ear, sinus, urinary tract) are just as effective with fewer side effects and better compliance.

BEWARE OF THE "ANTE-DIAGNOSIS"

One major error that some doctors make can pose a great danger to patients. I call this critical judgment lapse the "Ante-diagnosis." Some doctors will quickly jump to a diagnostic conclusion based on one particular initial impression. Having come to this premature conclusion, the doctor will then take any clues from the examination and tests and mold them to fit his or her initial diagnostic impression. It is not uncommon for the doctor to then ignore information that is inconsistent with the "Ante-diagnosis."

Why would a doctor jump to a conclusion? The explanation simply may be that the doctor is rushed and is trying to get the patient discharged or evaluated quickly. The doctor may not have enough time or knowledge to consider all diagnostic possibilities. This diagnostic lapse may simply come from an attitude the doctor develops about the patient in the initial moments of the doctor-patient encounter, the all important first impression. The consequences of an "Ante-diagnosis" can be disastrous as the following example illustrates.[14]

A middle-aged man with a history of high blood pressure is evaluated at an emergency room, because he developed severe upper back pain that seemed to travel to the chest. The man appeared to be extremely anxious as the emergency room doctor evaluated him. The chest X ray and electrocardiogram were normal, two important tests to help arrive at a diagnosis in someone stricken with these symptoms. The man was sent home with a prescription for a sedative.

The man returned to the emergency room the next morning still suffering from severe back pain. Again he appeared quite anxious to his family doctor who evaluated him. However, when a patient returns to an emergency room within a day, that in itself is a clue that something serious might be brewing. The family doctor reaffirmed that the electrocardiogram and chest X ray were normal and did no further investigation as he too had concluded the man was experiencing an anxiety attack. The other diagnosis was "viral syndrome," a diagnosis any patient should immediately be suspicious of since it often means the doctor does not know what is wrong, but wants to send you home quickly.

That evening the man's wife returned home after stepping out and found her husband lying on the floor, confused and wet from having urinated in his pants. After phoning her family doctor, still he stuck to his "ante-diagnosis" and assumed the problem was anxiety! He told the wife to place him in bed and call again in an hour. At this point, it should have been clear to the woman that her husband needed emergency care regardless of what her doctor was telling her. Never assume a doctor is correct when what he or she says or does defies common sense or your gut instinct.

By the time the man arrived at the emergency room, he was in shock from a ruptured aortic aneurysm, a fatal illness if the diagnosis is missed and treatment is delayed. The man died needlessly, even though the emergency doctor did mention aortic aneurysm as a possible diagnosis when the man was first evaluated.

Both doctors leaped to the diagnosis of anxiety because the man appeared to be so. Serious illness commonly causes anxiety, confusion, combativeness, restlessness and irritability. In this man, the adrenaline surge he likely was experiencing from the catastrophic illness that was brewing might have contributed to his anxious demeanor and appearance. Some people simply become anxious when they are ill and do not know what is wrong. Despite several good reasons to exclude the possibility of an aneurysm with a simple CAT scan, they jumped to an "ante-diagnosis" based on an impression about the man seeming anxious. Any management thereafter would be tailored to that premature diagnosis, even after the man was confused and very ill while lying on the floor. Common sense should always prevail in accepting a diagnosis, even if it is only the patient's family that has it.

USEFUL WEB SITES

http://www.ahcpr.gov/qual/errorsix.htm
(The Agency for Healthcare Research and Quality offers information on healthcare outcomes, quality, cost, errors, use and access.)

http://www.ama-assn.org/ama/pub/category3457.html
(The American Medical Association Health Information page provides timely health and medical information to consumers.)

http://www.medem.com/medlb/medlb_entry.cfm
(Medem's Medical Library holds a full range of patient education information from their partner medical societies.)

http://www.aap.org
(The American Academy of Pediatrics' Web site has up-to-date information on child healthcare for pediatricians and consumers/parents.)

http://www.aap.org/policy/re9751.html
(This site holds AAP's document titled "Prevention of Medication Errors in the Pediatric Inpatient Setting.")

http://ashp.com/bestpractices/medmis/guide/preventing.pdf
(This site has the American Society of Health-System Pharmacists' document titled "Preventing Medication Errors in Hospitals.")

http://www.iom.edu
(The Institute of Medicine offers timely information concerning health and science policy to government, corporations and the public.)

DANGER #3
INEPT AND UNSUITABLE SPECIALISTS

Jerry's crushing chest pain seemed to ease up the moment he saw the cardiologist arrive in the ER. The emergency doctor told him the heart specialist would inject a clot-dissolving drug to stop his massive heart attack. The medication would remove that "truckload of elephants" from his chest. Jerry was determined to recover for his three young children, but Jerry's faith in this specialist would soon turn to shock and disappointment.

Specialist care is a key aspect of emergency care. Emergency room doctors are jacks-of-all-trades and cannot possibly have expertise in treating every medical problem. ER physicians call upon the experience and proficiency of specialists when an illness or injury is severe or complex. A plastic surgeon, for instance, might be called to the emergency room to repair a disfiguring laceration, an orthopedic surgeon to set a badly broken bone. In addition, specialists are called in to treat patients and admit them into the hospital: a cardiologist might treat a man suffering from a heart attack in the ER, then have him admitted to the hospital for further care, while a surgeon would evaluate and decide to admit a patient with possible appendicitis.

Who decides which specialist to call? A pre-determined emergency room on-call schedule of doctors is set up at every hospital. Any specialists willing (or required by the hospital administration in order to retain hospital privileges) to take night calls will be placed on the twenty-four-hours/seven-days-a-week schedule. Competence and compassion are not, unfortunately, prerequisites to be a specialist. Since every hospital roster has both good and bad specialists in each field, quality of care ranges from inept and callous to expert and devoted. Jerry's specialist care would prove to be blatantly bad.

"Damn it! Where's the tPA?" the cardiologist yelled.

"We'll have the medication here in a minute," the nurse explained.

"I told the ER doctor to have it ready!"

"You asked for streptokinase on the telephone," the nurse snapped back.

"You're lying. You are all incompetent!" the cardiologist raged.

The cardiologist stormed into the cardiac treatment room and verbally abused the emergency doctor in front of the patient. Attempts to calm the specialist were unsuccessful as Jerry gasped for a full breath and stared in disbelief.

Soon the cardiologist became frenzied and out of control. He demanded the emergency doctor leave the cardiac room. Jerry clutched his chest when the specialist sprang at the emergency doctor and shoved him back a few steps. Concerned that the combative scene might cause a fatal heart rhythm in the patient, the emergency doctor left Jerry's room. That specialist put Jerry's life in danger with his inappropriate and anxiety causing behavior. Jerry did not know this could have been avoided had the emergency staff been able to call in a cardiologist they knew was compassionate and competent.

Most specialist incompetence is not as obvious as shown in the cases of Patricia's miscarriage or Jerry's heart attack experience. Inept specialist care is usually subtle enough that only nurses or doctors are able to recognize it and consists of: poor surgical skill or medical judgment; performing unnecessary surgery or procedures; delayed care in which patients are forced to wait hours to days for final treatment. Incredibly, specialist care might be delayed even during life-threatening medical crises! Deficient or faulty diagnosis and treatment by specialists can have three basic consequences for patients:
1. Delays and inconvenience
2. Needless suffering/disability
3. Loss of life or limb

DOCTOR DELAYS AND INCONVENIENCE

Many specialists resist coming to the hospital when summoned even though they are obligated to be on call to treat emergency room patients. They may use several tactics to unburden themselves of what they consider onerous duty. Perhaps the most common tactic is intimidation of the emergency physician with remarks such as "Do you know what time it is?" or "Can't this wait?" or "This is something you should be able to do." A second tactic is "turfing" the patient, which means passing the buck with comments like: "Transfer the patient" or "I don't see Medicare patients" or "I won't be able to get there for a few hours so get someone else" or "I don't have expertise in that area." These are the common responses, but they are not always phrased so politely.

This reluctance on the part of specialists to treat emergency room patients is most evident when the patient is uninsured or on public assistance, because there will be little or no payment for care rendered. Specialists, in fact, have grown resistant to treating even insured ER patients! The reason: they believe insurance reimbursement is too low.

At times, some specialists simply do not answer a beeper page from the hospital emergency room staff.[15]

For many of the same reasons, radiologists resist coming to the hospital ER to interpret an X ray or CAT scan. In a community hospital, the emergency doctor might be forced to rely on his or her own interpretation of a crucial X ray or on the opinion of the technician who is not licensed to make diagnoses. In a university hospital, an inexperienced radiology resident might make the final reading of a crucial X ray or CAT scan, leaving much room for error. As more radiologists use technology to allow transmission of X-ray images from hospitals directly to their homes, this particular specialist dilemma should be solved.

Consider the following examples of treatment delays and inconvenience to patients:

- A carpenter falls from a ladder and injures his neck. The emergency doctor isn't sure, but thinks he sees a subtle neck fracture on the X ray so he telephones the on-call radiologist. The radiologist refuses to come in to review the X rays. "You should be able to read a simple X ray," the radiologist says. Despite being paid a high salary to review all X rays, he would not come in promptly to review the films and help to confirm or exclude a possibly serious spine injury.

- A teenager breaks his ankle while playing football and because an orthopedic specialist cannot be persuaded to come in, his ankle is merely wrapped in the emergency room. He must make another long trip to an orthopedic clinic three days later to have a cast put on the ankle. His parents have no health insurance.

- A dog's teeth tear into a toddler's lip. After a four hour wait to be seen by the emergency room doctor, a hungry and cranky baby must wait an additional two hours until a plastic surgeon arrives from home to stitch the lip.

NEEDLESS SUFFERING/DISABILITY

Medical mistakes often lead to needless suffering or disability. While bizarre behavior on the part of specialists, like Patricia's and Jerry's experience, is a less common form of inept care, inexperience is probably the most frequent cause of avoidable treatment errors. When medical students or doctors-in-training are the "specialists" called upon to suture your wound or set your broken bone or treat your heart attack, mistakes will be plentiful. At teaching hospitals, inexperienced doctors are often unsupervised when treating emergency room patients and errors inevitably occur. Consider the following cases of physician inexperience leading to catastrophic consequences.

Not Just Another Case of Food Poisoning

An elderly man who lives at a nursing home is sent to the emergency department after vomiting a few times and appearing slightly dehydrated. A doctor-in-training who is on emergency room rotation assesses the man. The man has a fever of 101 degrees, looks a little dry and has a "soft" abdomen when the doctor presses on the lower right side. There is no reflexive muscle tensing typical of appendicitis. His urine test and white blood cell count, a measure of infection and inflammation, are within normal limits. Diagnosis: food poisoning. He gets two bags of intravenous fluids and is sent back to the home. The next day the elderly man returns to the emergency room, because he spiked a high fever, became confused and continued to vomit. He died the next week from complications of a ruptured appendix. The young doctor who initially examined him was unaware that the elderly frequently lack muscle tensing in the abdomen even in the presence of serious abdominal diseases.

Hidden Hand Damage

An electrician slices his hand with a utility knife and with the blood gushing, goes to a teaching hospital to get the "best" care. The emergency doctor is too busy to see him and calls a surgeon-in-training to care for the man's cut hand. The young doctor glances at the deep cut, happy to have a chance to practice his suturing technique. He asks the electrician to bend all fingers and the man complies. "Looks like everything's okay," the doctor says with a smile and stitches up the cut in the man's hand. A few weeks later, the electrician goes to a hand specialist, because two fingers on the hand he cut could not bend. In fact, two tendons were sliced by the utility knife, but remained connected by only a few fibers. The tendons completely separated when the man began moving his fingers again. The surgeon-in-training completely missed the deeper injury.

Consider the subtleties of aggressive versus conservative treatment. Sometimes it is better medical practice to watch and wait, while at other times an immediate procedure or surgery is appropriate and perhaps lifesaving. Many cardiologists routinely prefer an aggressive approach to treating patients with newly diagnosed chest pains (unstable angina). These patients will probably undergo heart catheterization (angiogram), a potentially dangerous procedure in which wires are threaded through a leg artery into the heart. Dye is injected to delineate the arteries that feed the heart and to check for blockages. Other heart specialists might first try a conservative approach to treat stable patients, using only medications and waiting to see if the chest pains cease.

Heart specialists who advocate aggressive treatment might say they want to know exactly what is going on with a patient's heart and elect to do the invasive procedure. It seems to make sense. However, several studies have shown that a conservative approach is often safer. Major heart studies with names like OASIS, TIMI IIIB and VAN-QWISH have found that an aggressive approach of heart catheterization within two days of chest pains can have a higher ultimate death rate than an approach with fewer procedures and waiting to see how a patient responds to medications.[16] Clearly, an individual patient approach is appropriate with consideration of risks versus benefits before proceeding to risky procedures.

Greed can place patients at risk as well. Earning more money can be a powerful motivator for some specialists to perform unnecessary procedures. A few specialists will do avoidable angiograms, intestinal "scopes" or surgeries which only a nurse or doctor can recognize as unnecessary. Some people might even admire these doctors' aggressive approach, viewing it as "pro-active." The pain from these avoidable procedures, however, is significant and serious complications from surgery and invasive procedures commonly occur. Many patients will never know that the procedure done on them was not necessary. Conversely, patients might never know that a delay in their care—perhaps an immediate procedure or quicker response by a specialist—could have helped avert suffering and disability.

Life or Death Decisions Gone Awry

The emergency physician has difficulty placing a breathing tube into the windpipe of a woman who is gasping for air. The place: A community hospital emergency room. The time: 3:00 A.M. The covering anesthesiologist must be notified at home, then he or she must dress and drive fifteen minutes or so to get to the hospital and assist the emergency physician. There is only one problem: Brain cells begin to die after only four minutes of oxygen deprivation and the breathing tube will not be properly inserted for nearly twenty minutes. Teaching hospitals, by contrast, have anesthesiologists or nurse anesthetists present in the hospital twenty-four hours every day. The woman with breathing problems ultimately dies. Could she have been saved with the more immediately available expert care at a larger, teaching hospital?

At a community hospital, a pediatrician refuses to come in to the emergency department to help the lone emergency room doctor care for a critically ill toddler. "I live sixty minutes away" or "Transfer the baby to a university hospital" are common responses from some specialists. This means the baby does not get the "expert care" of a pediatrician to double-check the baby's treatment plan as implemented by the ER doctor. Moreover, the lone emergency doctor and few nurses must continue to see other patients, leaving the seriously ill toddler with a bare minimum of supervision. If the child's condition suddenly deteriorated, a young life might be lost. If a vital medication was not adjusted, not given soon enough or not administered in proper dosage, that error could make the difference between a child dying that day or living a full life.

A life and death delay occurs when a car accident victim is brought unconscious to a community hospital. She needs emergency surgery to control internal bleeding in the abdomen and/or chest. The emergency doctor does all that can be done to stabilize the patient. The only way to save her life is immediate surgery to tie off the bleeding arteries or veins. The surgeon arrives from home several minutes later, but too late to save her. By the time the woman is wheeled up to the operating room, she has no pulse or blood pressure. Could more immediate surgery have saved that woman's life or were her injuries just too severe?

A man who is having a massive heart attack believes he went to the right university hospital—one large enough to have the technology to save his life. Surprisingly, the man does not receive emergency balloon angioplasty, the best available treatment to stop his massive heart attack. Instead, he gets clot-dissolving medication, a treatment that is less effective than scraping out the blood clot from the heart-feeding artery. The reason: It is 3:00 A.M. and the cardiology staff at this teaching hospital will not come into the hospital at all hours of the night. He had no way of knowing that another teaching hospital a few minutes drive away offers this life-saving procedure at any hour of the day.

It is frightening to think that patients might needlessly suffer or lose life or limb because a specialist does not promptly tend to their medical needs. Your life can truly depend upon being taken to the right hospital emergency room at the right time. Forewarned is forearmed. Learn the pros and cons of the different emergency care facilities in your area. When sudden illness or injury strike, you will know where best to go for your particular problem.

HOW CAN I SOLVE THE SPECIALIST DILEMMA?

Why are specialists who are on emergency room call reluctant to come in to treat a patient? The reasons are basic: overwork and underpay lead to apathy. If you were about to have dinner with your family after a fourteen-hour workday, would you want to rush out the door, hungry and tired? Your desire to leave the house is even less, knowing you may get paid little, if anything, for your efforts.

What's more, just because a specialist does come to the hospital to treat an emergency room patient, it does not guarantee quality care. Every hospital has mediocre and inept specialist physicians who might be on emergency room call the night you or your loved one arrives at a hospital. What can you do to maximize your chances for quality specialist care?

Suggestions for Quality Specialist Care:

1. *Go To a Teaching Hospital Emergency Room*: At teaching hospitals, specialists in most fields are available in the hospital twenty-four hours each day. These specialists can be in the emergency room within minutes in an emergency situation. The **caveat**: That specialist who treats you might actually be a doctor-in-training with little experience thus far in the specialty. For instance, the orthopedist who places a cast on your broken leg might be a second-year resident training in the field of orthopedics. He or she might do a fine or inept job—it is unpredictable. The doctor who restarts your heart with a pacemaker might be a first-year "Fellow" who just started subspecialty training in cardiology or even a less experienced resident. Patients can request that an experienced specialist be called to treat a more complex problem at teaching hospitals. If an "Attending" (completed training, more experienced) specialist will not come to the emergency room, ask the emergency staff to call another one. If that fails, request that the Chief or Senior Resident supervise or provide care for your problem. Inexperience can also have serious consequences for repair of cuts, especially those on the hands and face. Community hospitals, on the other hand, usually do not have doctors-in-training. The specialist called to treat your ailment will be, at the least, one who has completed training (an "Attending Physician").

2. *Go To a Hospital Emergency Room at Which Your Family Doctor Has Privileges*: Ask your family doctor to guide your treatment in the emergency room (via telephone or in person). If you need a cardiologist for a heart problem or an orthopedist for a broken bone, your family doctor can recommend an experienced specialist. Emergency staff will then not be obligated by policy to use the possibly unpredictable specialist on call. The **caveat**: Your trusty family doctor might recommend a specialist who is more inept than the one on call for the emergency room. Doctors recommend other physicians based on friendship, style of practice, familiarity and unspoken agreements of "You send me patients and I will send you patients." Just because your family doctor (whom you trust, hopefully) chooses a specialist, it is no guarantee *that* doctor is the most skilled. How then can you get the best man or woman for the job of caring for you? The answer might be right in front of you.

3. *Ask Emergency Room Staff Which Specialist They Would Use For Their Own Care*: Talk to several nurses and doctors. Inquire about which specialist they would use for their own mother. Get a few opinions. Some staff might be reluctant to give out specific names since there is a predetermined call schedule in the ER. Giving out names might be construed as "stealing" patients away from the doctor on call or indirectly bad-mouthing a specialist. There is another way to look at it: patients get the best possible care when treated by the most competent specialists. Isn't that the purpose of the emergency room? Indeed, emergency room nurses and doctors routinely see all specialists in action so they know who is pleasant, who is skilled and who is inept. What can you do if emergency workers clam up when you ask for their personal opinion about a specialist? Ask the doctor or nurse in a friendly, indirect fashion. If Dr. Smith is on call for cardiology, for example, ask the following: "Doc, would you use Dr. Smith for your heart attack?" At the least, you will get some limited response such as a facial expression or eye-rolling—enough to answer your question. Once you get the name of a quality specialist, "request" that doctor by name. That enables the emergency staff to bypass the on-call schedule of specialists. Bear in mind, this is research that can be done before it becomes necessary, as in selecting an appropriate emergency facility. Begin now to compile a list of recommended specialists who practice in your area.

4. *Call Another Specialist*: If the first specialist who is called by the ER staff is hard to reach or cannot come in promptly for an emergency,

request that a second specialist be called. Ask for a recommendation. Another **caveat**: If a specialist is too eager to perform a procedure or operation that is elective (not immediately lifesaving), you should get a second opinion from another specialist. If you do not have confidence in the specialist who cares for you in the emergency department, you can turn down or put on hold his or her recommendations and try to get a second opinion.

5. *Ask To Be Transferred To Another Hospital:* Many community and rural hospitals do not have all specialties immediately available. Sometimes it is difficult to contact specialists due to holidays, vacations or operating room duty. Furthermore, it is not uncommon for specialists to have insufficient training for certain medical problems. Many orthopedists, for instance, do not have expert training for treating serious hand injuries. In such a case, you would want to be seen by a hand surgeon, usually either an orthopedist or plastic surgeon who has additional training and expertise in hand injuries. If emergency room staff tell you the on-call specialist will be hard to reach, is not responding to a page in a timely fashion or is less than qualified to treat your specific problem, request a transfer to a university hospital so you can get the expert care you need.

6. *Ask Whether Your Treatment Can Wait:* As a last resort, ask the emergency doctor if you can wait to have your medical problem treated by a specialist in a day or two. You can then seek care from a specialist with whom you are familiar. Not every broken bone needs a full cast immediately, an appropriate splint will do fine for a short period of time. Not every twinge of chest pain requires an urgent consultation with a cardiologist. Specialty care for less serious injury or illness can wait a day or more. Whether it is a broken bone or sudden illness, if you trust the emergency physician, then heed his or her advice as to whether definitive care can wait or not. If you are unsure, call your family doctor to get another opinion.

DANGER #4
BELIEVING ALL DOCTORS
ARE CREATED EQUAL

Consider these scenarios: A friend recommends that you to go to an internist rather than a plastic surgeon to have a gash on your face stitched. That's odd, you think. A relative suggests you take your sick child to an adult stomach specialist and not a pediatrician. You scratch your head, puzzled. Your spouse insists that you take your father to a general surgeon and not a cardiologist to check on his heart condition. These scenarios are far-fetched; they would never happen!

Amazingly, this is precisely what can happen when you visit an emergency room! Who is that physician who treats you? What is his or her training background? If you believe all emergency room doctors are about the same, you are mistaken. Emergency physician training and experience are as variable as the weather. Consider these cases:

CASE 1

It was a typically busy day in the emergency room: two patients with heart attacks, two with breathing trouble, an assortment of pains and the usual injuries. The lone emergency room doctor, amidst the tumult at this community hospital, began to suture a woman's lip laceration. With one eye focused on the man experiencing seizures and one ear listening for rhythm changes on a beeping heart monitor, the doctor quickly stitched the cut together. "Five stitches," the physician said with a smile as he placed the needles in the disposal and raced off to check on other patients.

When her family doctor removed the stitches a few days later, the woman looked at her lip in the mirror and shrieked. Her ordeal was not over. It had just begun.

She turned away from the mirror, mortified at what she saw. Part of her cut involved the dark-pink part of the lip on which lipstick is worn. If this "vermilion border" is not aligned perfectly, it heals with an irregular notch in the smooth lip outline, comparable to not aligning the edges of a wallpaper pattern. Why did this cosmetic calamity happen? To understand the reason, the woman would need to know about the professional background of the emergency doctor who sutured her lip.

CASE 2

An elderly man arrived at a university hospital emergency department complaining of dizziness and mild breathing difficulty. The nurse measured his blood pressure: "eighty systolic," which is very low and a likely cause for his dizziness. The emergency doctor watched the electrocardiogram machine write its squiggly script on the heat-sensitive paper. "No indication it's a heart attack," the doctor said. Amidst the machine beeps and patient groans, he briefly listened with his stethoscope to the man's lungs. "Sounds clear." The doctor ordered a quart of intravenous fluids to be given rapidly. "Another life saved," he muttered as he sped away to the next patient.

The elderly man lay on the stretcher confused and afraid. After a while, he pulled on his intravenous line then tried to jump off the stretcher. Intravenous fluids briskly poured into his vein from the still attached tube. By now, his breathing rate had doubled. His pink lips and fingernails turned blue minutes before the nurse sounded a Code Blue alert. The emergency doctor, who had only glanced at him once in four hours, bolted to his bedside.

When the doctor arrived at the elderly man's bedside, a medical student had started CPR. Each time the student compressed the man's breastbone, the student felt the cracking and crunching of breaking ribs. The physician placed a breathing tube into the man's windpipe, releasing a geyser of frothy pink fluid—a sign the man was suffering from severe heart failure. They injected several drugs into his stiff body. Nothing helped.

The patient was dead. The man was mistakenly given fluids to increase his low blood pressure when in fact it was heart failure that caused the low blood pressure. Treatment should have included eliminating water from his body, not giving extra fluid. The intravenous fluid led to his rapid demise. To understand why this man died, his grieving children would need to know about the training background of the treating emergency physician.

CASE 3

A worried mother rushed her child to the community hospital emergency room at three o'clock in the morning when the little girl spiked a fever of 105.4 degrees. The baby had been taking amoxicillin for one week for an ear infection and the original fever had normalized two days before. The fever had returned and the mother was worried because her little one had not been playful since yesterday.

The ER nurse walked over to the doctor's call room, knocked loudly on the door and awakened the emergency doctor from a deep but short sleep. "I have a patient for you," she whispered. She heard tossing in bed.

The doctor struggled to focus his eyes on his watch. He grimaced and asked, "Why do the patients have to be insomniacs? What is it that's so important at 3:00 A.M.?"

"Don't worry, doc, it's a simple one. Sounds like otitis treatment failure," the nurse answered.

The weary-eyed doctor emerged from his call room, his eyes burning from the bright corridor lights. He tightened the knot on his green scrub pants and was still yawning when he arrived at the bedside. Performing a rapid, one-minute examination, the doctor asked three direct questions, interrupting the mother's concerned comments, and then explained that it was probably a treatment failure of the baby's ear infection. While the physician scribbled a prescription for a different antibiotic, the mother wondered why the doctor neglected to ask about her baby's eating and behavior changes, like the pediatrician always asked. The doctor thought, *Well-behaved, quiet baby. At least that's one advantage of the early morning hour.*

The physician handed the mother the prescription. The doctor returned to his call room to sleep. The baby went home to die.

The training background of the emergency physician who sent the child home would be of interest to the anguished mother who lost her baby. The baby actually had meningitis, an infection of the brain that probably spread there from her ear infection. This serious infection went unsuspected by the doctor for several reasons. First, he was in a rush to get back to sleep so he hurried his questioning, examination and thought processes. The second reason relates to training background, a common thread to these three tragic cases—the woman with a lip laceration sutured improperly, the elderly man who died from fluid overload and the child with a serious infection that was missed.

Going to an emergency room for medical care can at times be likened to calling a carpenter to fix a leaky pipe. A surgeon who rarely studied electrocardiograms during five years of training might be managing your heart attack or reassuring you that your chest pain is not a heart problem. The person in a green scrub suit who stitches the cut on your face at a teaching hospital will likely be a medical student or intern (first year doctor-in-training) who "saw one, did one, taught one," an unfortunate but true medical aphorism. An internist (who is doing specialty training in gastroenterology) might send your baby home from a community hospital ER telling you not to worry, but not telling you that he or she has treated few if any babies since medical school.

Just what is the training background of emergency room doctors? What are the qualifications of those who treat you in an emergency department? In fact, not every health provider who dons a white coat is a doctor. And many emergency room doctors are neither sufficiently experienced nor properly trained for the job of providing urgent care.

EMERGENCY ROOM DOCTORS

Senior Attending Physicians

To serve as a senior (attending) physician in the emergency room, a physician must have at least three years of residency training under his or her belt. This might mean completed training in internal medicine or family practice or as yet uncompleted training in surgery, pediatrics or the specialty of emergency medicine.

Does completion of training guarantee competence in the emergency room? Absolutely not! It is unfortunate that many physicians who are likely to practice in the emergency room setting are not taught during training many of the skills needed for good emergency care. For instance, few internists (Internal Medicine training, general care doctors) can confidently manage breathing crises, orthopedic injuries, eye problems, pediatric illness or gynecologic problems upon completion of their prescribed three years of training. The specialties of family practice and emergency medicine train jacks-of-all-trades. These physicians spend short stints learning internal medicine, surgery, pediatrics, obstetrics and other fields necessary for emergency or primary care. Some would argue these jacks-of-all-trades know something about many illnesses, but are masters of nothing.

Many surgeons have no expertise and little practical experience managing commonplace medical illness such as diabetes, heart attacks, emphysema and heart failure. Yet many doctors trained as general surgeons serve as senior physicians and treat these medical illnesses in emergency departments. Pediatricians staff emergency rooms only in larger teaching hospitals with separate pediatric emergency care areas.

There are great variations in skills and diagnostic abilities among physicians, but at least attending physicians have completed formal training in their respective fields. If these physicians practice emergency medicine on a full-time basis, they will ultimately become more experienced and more capable. Incredibly, many attending physicians' skills are learned or perfected on the job in emergency rooms, sometimes at patients' expense!

Teaching hospital emergency rooms are swarming with inexperienced doctors. Interns, residents and fellows are relatively inexperienced doctors. Interns know little or nothing about hands-on patient care. Residents are doctors in the second through fifth years of training, depending on the specialty. At this point in their careers, most of these doctors-in-training generally have a simplistic understanding of disease based on textbook descriptions of classic symptoms. They do not yet have enough experience to understand that less typical signs and symptoms of disease that deviate from textbooks happen the majority of the time.

Fellows have completed three to five years of residency training and are gaining expertise in specialty fields such as plastic surgery, cardiology, gastroenterology or others. Each level of doctor training brings with it new knowledge, but more responsibility. Similar to training in any field, *inexperience* and mistakes go hand in hand. It has been said that, "The true point to a residency is to avoid *repeating* preventable errors." The training of young doctors is certainly a vital part of our healthcare system. Learning with close supervision can enhance the training experience without compromising patient care. Thrusting inexperienced workers into emergency rooms to learn by trial and error means mistakes will be made. For the ill or injured individuals seeking urgent care, there is simply too high a price to be paid for inadequate physician training and preparedness.

An unfortunate paradox of the teaching hospital is while young doctors and other healthcare providers must actively ask for help in order to learn and grow as professionals, requesting guidance or assistance is often considered a sign of weakness or incompetence. Moreover, if an inexperienced healthcare provider does not know or recognize early and subtle signs of a serious illness, he or she will not know when to insist on getting help. Since senior physicians do not examine many patients, a significant number of sick people showing atypical symptoms or in the early stages of serious illness will not get proper treatment from the inexperienced healthcare providers who perform the initial examinations. An inexperienced doctor, for instance, might be quick to diagnose a stomach virus in a baby who is irritable, has fever and vomits. An astute, experienced clinician knows these symptoms can be an early sign of illness such as meningitis or serious intestinal problems. To some inexperienced providers, back pain is usually a muscle strain problem, while a seasoned physician immediately tries to exclude serious conditions such as heart attack, aortic aneurysm, pneumonia or kidney stones.

Inexperience is not limited to doctors-in-training who need closer supervision. Every emergency room employs "moonlighters"—attending physicians who do ER work part-time or doctors who are still in training (senior Residents or Fellows). These physicians work fifty to eighty hours weekly in their chosen specialty and occasionally work the emergency room just to earn extra money or to gain patient care experience. Sensibly, doctors-in-training are not allowed to deliver babies in the delivery room nor operate in the operating room just to earn extra cash or gain experience. Why should these inexperienced physicians be able to work on the front lines—the emergency room—where life or death decisions are made? An inexperienced young doctor or exhausted moonlighter with expertise in an unrelated specialty one day might be managing your varied and urgent medical needs. These are the options with which you might be faced when you seek help at an emergency room. You would not allow a carpenter to fix a water-main leak in your house. Would you want a general surgeon to treat your serious heart attack? For these reasons, it is vital that a patient ask who is treating him or her and what the training is of that healthcare provider.

Other Healthcare Providers

Doctors are not the sole healthcare providers working in hospital emergency departments. As hospitals try to save money, they are replacing medical doctors with nurse practitioners or physician assistants, replacing registered nurses with medical or nurse assistants and are cutting clerical staff as well. Less skill and training equals lower wages the hospital must pay. Providers such as physician assistants, nurse practitioners, medical students and students in other healthcare fields might be working at an emergency department near you. Paramedics often assist doctors with care of critically ill patients, particularly when the emergency room is shorthanded and busy. In fact, research done five years ago found that about one in twenty-five people who were evaluated in America's emergency departments were seen by either a nurse practitioner or physician assistant. They cared for patients suffering from possibly serious illnesses such as chest pain, abdominal pain, fever, lacerations and severe headaches, not just minor ailments. The number of nurse practitioners and physician assistants treating emergency department patients probably has increased since 1995.

Nurse Practitioners

The distinction between a physician and other healthcare providers is an important one. Nurse practitioners are nurses who did additional training in treating everyday illness. They diagnose disease, write prescriptions and often serve as primary healthcare providers. While nurse practitioners can have excellent (or poor) clinical judgment similar to doctors, they have considerably less training and experience than a seasoned doctor.

Physician Assistants

Physician assistants also have far less training than medical doctors and are required by law to work directly under a physician's direction. An important component of the care provided by physician assistants, nurse practitioners and students, as well as a significant aspect of their learning, is going over patient problems with an experienced physician. That physician should also be available to examine patients who have more complex illnesses. Unfortunately, that supervision is often comprised of a one-minute conversation about a particular patient without the senior physician ever examining the patient. There are many instances when supervision is nonexistent, because it is just too busy or senior physicians are neglecting their teaching duties.

Returning to the three patient stories discussed earlier: The doctor who left a jagged border on the woman's lip was an internist with little minor or plastic surgical experience. It was a doctor trained in surgery who filled that elderly man's lungs with more fluid, leading to his death. Believe it or not, the doctor who sent that sick baby home to die was completing training in adult gastroenterology! The only time he treated babies was when he moonlighted in the emergency room, was never formally trained in baby care and rarely read or concerned himself with the latest information on pediatric ailments. Clearly, whether in university hospitals or smaller community hospitals, the healthcare provider who cares for you or your loved one at an emergency room may not be the best person for the job.

FINDING A QUALITY DOCTOR/HEALTHCARE PROVIDER IN THE ER

The Josiah Macy, Jr. Foundation released a report confirming a frightening fact that every practicing emergency physician and nurse already knows: Many doctors who staff our nation's emergency rooms are poorly qualified and lack the necessary skills for the job. It is shocking that doctors who treat patients, many of whom are on the brink of death or in dire straits, are poorly trained for the job! What are the general functions of an emergency room doctor? Along with the ability to handle demanding and stressful work, ER doctors must have the skills to:

- Stabilize patients who are critically ill and might die within minutes. This requires many procedural skills, instant decision-making ability and specialized knowledge.
- Distinguish between potentially serious illness and those that will get better on their own.
- Treat people who are in cardiac arrest.
- Care for children with serious injuries or illness.
- Alleviate severe pain.
- Treat patients with serious psychiatric illness.
- Stabilize and care for those strung out on illegal drugs, suffering alcoholic dependency or drug overdoses, violent patients, victims of violence and children who have been abused—situations that are frequently emotionally draining on physicians and nurses.
- Treat gunshot wound and stabbing victims.
- Reassure patients and family members or console them.
- Inform patients about what to do and what signs to look for if their conditions deteriorate.
- Admit patients into the hospital, if needed.
- Arrange for specialist care or consultation.
- Perform many minor surgical procedures such as suturing cuts, draining abscesses and placing special intravenous lines into large veins in the chest, neck or thigh.
- Care for patients with varied problems including those involving the eyes, genitals and reproductive organs.
- Deliver babies.

These functions might sound straightforward, but they require instantaneous decisions and complicated skills. An emergency doctor must intubate patients with serious breathing compromise, administer potent drugs in an eye-blink and must have vast medical knowledge to pinpoint in an instant which of ten different illnesses is the likely cause for a patient not being able to breathe, for instance. They must also understand the differences in diagnosing and treating illness in babies and children.

Moonlighters, more than other emergency room doctors, tend to lack key skills and training. These physicians have unrelated or limited specialty training (gastroenterology, orthopedics, surgery, etc.) and work in the emergency room part-time to earn extra money. The director of a major New York City trauma emergency department stated in the Macy report that some physicians working in emergency rooms were not taught how to treat a heart attack, resuscitate a child or treat bleeding. Yet these are the doctors on whom you might depend to save your own or a parent's or child's life!

Patients are needlessly dying, according to the Macy report, because many emergency physicians know less than paramedics about treating critical illnesses. Why are inadequately trained physicians working on the front lines of our nation's emergency rooms? What compels a healthcare system to compromise the most important aspect of its medical care? First, there are not enough well trained emergency physicians to go around, particularly in rural and community hospitals. Second, emergency physician burnout is rampant, because of high stress and overwork on the job. Third, emergency room directors hire moonlighters to work shifts, because they are a source of cheaper labor and they are willing to work less desirable weekend and night shifts.

The Macy Foundation report called for the establishment of minimum qualifications for doctors and nurses who work in emergency departments, with special attention to moonlighting physicians. You might find in your local emergency room medical students, young doctors-in-training (interns and residents), unsupervised physicians assistants and nurse practitioners, inadequately trained moonlighters, and primary care doctors such as internists who are fresh out of training. All of these providers might be inexperienced and unskilled in front-line, urgent care, particularly if working alone at a community hospital.

Lack of skills is not limited to doctors. Some hospitals, for instance, are forced to hire ER charge nurses who have no critical care experience, simply because they can find no others with experience to take the high-stress positions. Nurses are considered the backbone of emergency departments. If they lack key skills or knowledge to assist doctors, lives can be lost when procedures are delayed or performed improperly. As hospitals hire less expensive medical assistants to replace nurses because of budget cuts, less skilled workers may lead to the reduced quality of patients' care. Consider the consequences when a doctor needs assistance placing a breathing tube into a patient's windpipe. If the nurse or medical assistant does not know the maneuver, called "cricoid pressure" and which enables the doctor to see the windpipe more clearly, valuable time is lost. Patients might die when emergency nurses are unfamiliar with the use of defibrillation paddle equipment, causing a delay in jump-starting a patient's failed heart. Even if only a two minute delay, those two minutes can be the difference between success and failure, life or death.

Until minimum standards are implemented, what can you do to avoid receiving inadequate care by emergency room healthcare providers? You cannot change hospital staff procedures, but you can improve your chances for quality care with simple information and pre-planning. The first rule, at the risk of being redundant, is to avoid the emergency room if at all possible. Seek medical care at your doctor's office whenever possible and before problems become serious. On the other hand, if you seek care too soon for problems that will get better on their own, your doctor will not be able to do much for you other than to give reassurance.

While familiarity is comforting and probably safer, too, predictability is nonexistent in the emergency room setting. Your family doctor, on the other hand, is familiar to you and you are (or should be) familiar to your doctor. Do not underestimate the importance of a doctor knowing your history, habits and personality. The emergency doctor knows little or nothing about you, your medical history or your normal state of health. Another key aspect of seeing a doctor in an office is that he or she is unlikely to be handling many other seriously ill patients while examining you. The emergency doctor probably is and will not be able to spend much time on your behalf.

If you cannot get an appointment with your family doctor or in the case of a true crisis, must rush to the emergency room, you most likely will not be able to choose the doctor or other provider who will oversee your ER care. If your family doctor cannot meet you at the emergency room, it will be the luck of the draw as to who picks up your chart to evaluate you. You can, however, judge him or her in the same way you would your family doctor. While the doctor or other care provider speaks to you, determine if he or she has a good bedside manner, makes sensible decisions, asks good questions, spends a reasonable amount of time with you based on how sick you are and communicates well.

FOUR KEY QUALITIES
IN EMERGENCY ROOM PHYSICIANS
OR OTHER HEALTHCARE PROVIDERS:

- Competence
- Reputation or expertise
- Compassion
- Communication skills and time spent with you

Competence

Competence is surely the most important quality and the one most difficult to judge, particularly in a hurried, one-time emergency room encounter. There are signs to look for and several questions you can ask the treating physician or provider. These answers will give you a rough measure of competence.

- What is your field of training? Skip the question about what medical school the doctor went to—it is meaningless.
- Have you completed training? If yes, how long have you practiced emergency medicine? Do you work full time as an emergency room doctor/provider or are you a moonlighter?
- Are you board-certified in your field of training? This means the doctor took and passed a standardized examination given to others in that specialty. The medical field takes it very seriously. Does it mean the doctor is definitely competent? Not necessarily, but it is a helpful method of assessment. The *Official ABMS Directory of Board Certified Medical Specialists* lists all certified physicians by specialty. You can find it at your local library or on the World Wide Web.
- Diligence and being thorough are also important qualities in a provider. If your caretaker calls for old records or previous electrocardiogram or other test results, that is a positive sign. Sound clinical judgment, unfortunately, is not something that can easily be taught to a doctor or other healthcare provider; however, it seems likely that the more experienced the doctor, the better judgment and clinical skills he or she will have.

Expertise

A physician's expertise can be measured in several ways: research done, papers published, teaching at a medical school or the number of operations performed. This type of expertise is more important if you are searching for a surgeon to do your heart bypass operation or for a kidney specialist to treat your unusual kidney disease. Expertise is also crucial in situations of life-threatening accidents, falls or gunshot wounds, serious illness in children and serious heart attacks. Successful treatment is dependent also upon a hospital having available the advanced technology and specialty care needed, as well as the doctor's individual skill and experience. If a person has a blood clot in the brain, for example, his life will be saved if a neurosurgeon promptly drills holes in the skull to drain the clot and release the pressure. In situations like this, the emergency doctor can only keep the patient alive by delaying deterioration until life-saving surgery is performed. Once again, there is no substitute for experience.

Compassion

A third quality you should look for in a physician/provider is compassion. Five minutes with a doctor or other care provider will tell you about his or her bedside manner—if you get that much time with an emergency doctor. Many emergency room doctors are compassionate, but it is unfortunate that time to spend with each patient is limited because of overcrowding.

Communication skills

Lastly, a physician's communication skills and the amount of time that doctor/provider spends with you is important. Does he or she explain things simply and reassure you and your family? Does he or she tell you the risks, advantages and disadvantages of performing tests or giving treatments? Does he or she discuss all possible options? Most importantly, does the doctor answer your questions and ask for your input in making decisions about your care? Consider how different a patient's decisions and outlook will be with these two very different physician approaches to the same situation:

1. "Ma'am, you're having a myocardial infarction which can kill you so I'm going to administer intravenous medicine to help save your life."
2. "You are having a relatively small heart attack, but you are quite stable and will be just fine. Here are your choices: clot-dissolving treatment which can help, but has possibly serious risks including ...or watch and wait using safer medications such as..."

Clearly, a patient will likely make different choices based on these two dissimilar approaches by the doctors.

If your emergency room doctor (or other provider) makes sense and instills confidence in you, then go with your gut feeling. If you are unhappy with the emergency doctor's approach or training background or if that doctor has not spent much time on your behalf, you have several options. First, have the emergency doctor confer with your family doctor before making an important decision. This communication is crucial so the emergency doctor can get key information about your medical history from the doctor who knows you best.

Another option you should be aware of is your right to request that an appropriate specialist such as a cardiologist or orthopedic surgeon consult on your behalf. If the doctor who evaluates you is only a physician-in-training or medical student, you can request that an emergency room Attending (senior) physician evaluate you in addition to the Resident. Unfortunately, you might not always be accommodated. With any healthcare provider who is not a senior physician, you should ask if that provider has discussed the case with a senior physician. You should also request that the senior physician examine you, speak with you and your family doctor and get more actively involved on your behalf.

A call into your family doctor to have him or her meet you at the emergency room can bypass the need for you to see the emergency doctor. Unfortunately, few family physicians are that devoted. This is particularly true if your doctor works out of a university hospital, in which case your doctor will wait for the emergency doctor or doctor-in-training (Resident) to evaluate you and then give him or her a call. Of course, if you are sure you know what kind of a specialist you need, i.e., cardiac, orthopedic, etc., and you have done your homework and have one or two recommended names, you can have the ER staff or a family member call and ask to have the specialist see you in the emergency room. This is dependent on your insurance coverage and also on whether the specialist has privileges at the particular hospital in which you find yourself. Again, pre-planning is key.

Ultimately, you might have no choice but to depend upon the treating emergency physician. Knowing the healthcare provider's training and expertise, as well as relying on your impressions, can help you decide whether or not to place your health in that individual's hands.

USEFUL WEB SITES

http://www.abms.org
(The American Board of Medical Specialities' Web site has a listing all of board certified members in the United States.)

http://www.ama-assn.org
(The American Medical Association's Web site has a wealth of information on health and well-being for consumers as well as current news and features like "Doctor Finder" and "Hospital Finder.")

http://www.health.state.ny.us/nysdoh/consumer/heart/homehear.htm
(New York State Health Department's information page on heart disease provides downloadable documents on a variety of issues.)

http://homearts.com/gh/health/03cardf1.htm
(This 1996 *Good Housekeeping* article lists names and profiles of the country's top doctors in heart and stroke treatment and care.)

DANGER #5
TRIAGE TRAVESTIES

A man leaned on the registration desk of the hospital emergency room, his two young children standing at his side. In heavily accented English, he told the clerk that he woke up three hours earlier with shoulder pain.

"Which shoulder hurts?" the desk clerk inquired.

"My left," he murmured, grimacing and clutching that shoulder.

"Did you fall, sir?" She looked up at his pale face.

"No, no. I felt it when I woke up," he answered, his hand pressing on the desk to support his weight.

The computer printer hammered out a chart listing his complaint as "shoulder pain." The triage nurse read it and stuffed it under a pile of charts as a minor orthopedic problem. Sitting between his children in the waiting room, the man clutched his head trying desperately to steady it. His children were giggling at pictures in a magazine when he collapsed and fell to the floor. People in the waiting area gaped. The man's children paced around the room pleading for help while their father's eyes bulged, teeth clenched and limbs flailed.

Their father was wheeled into the emergency department, oxygen mask over his mouth and nose, heart monitor leads pasted onto his chest, intravenous line in his arm. His blood pressure: sixty over thirty. Heart rate: thirty. He had a seizure because he was not getting enough oxygen and blood to his brain. Intravenous medication normalized his vital signs. The man had, in fact, suffered a heart attack. In his case, the shoulder pain was not a joint injury, but a less common manifestation of impending heart damage.

A heart attack can cause seemingly harmless symptoms like tooth pain, shoulder pain, indigestion, back pain, arm discomfort or even hiccups. An astute triage nurse might have recognized the man's pale color and difficulty standing as clues to more serious illness. He nearly died from this oversight. In his case, first impressions led to an inaccurate, quick conclusion and nearly resulted in a tragedy.

Immediate impressions in the emergency room are so important that an entire system of sorting urgently ill from not so ill patients, called triage, is based upon these quick assessments. The traditional setup of many emergency rooms is that of a small booth or room having a desk at its center and a blood pressure cuff, digital thermometer and blood-drawing tubes and needles alongside the desk. Seated in front of the desk is a specially trained nurse who quickly evaluates the patient, measures vital signs including temperature, blood pressure and pulse rate and determines if the problem is urgent or less pressing. "Urgent" is defined as an illness that might or will lead to loss of life or limb. Severe pain and bleeding also fall into the urgent category. Everything else can wait on a first-come, first-serve basis. Many emergency rooms have fine-tuned evaluation to include a separate fast-track section to treat those with less urgent problems like cuts, aches, sprains, minor fractures and colds.

It is troubling that many emergency rooms do not have an immediate triage area. A patient first registers with a desk clerk and gives out insurance and personal information. A chief complaint such as "cough" or "abdominal pain" is then recorded on the chart. The clerk has no formal medical training. Most clerks know phrases like "shortness of breath" or "asthma" or "chest pain" may indicate serious problems and when they hear them they immediately notify the triage nurse who then evaluates the patient. For other complaints, the patient is directed to the waiting area until the triage nurse gets to his or her chart for the screening evaluation. At busy times in the ER, the wait from time of registration until the screening evaluation by the triage nurse could be hours, at quiet times only minutes. Patients who arrive by ambulance go directly into the main emergency room eliminating the triage procedure.

What if the triage nurse has a wrong first impression? Worse yet, clerks frequently misjudge degree of illness or potential for crisis since they have no medical training. Yet at many emergency rooms, these clerks are on the front lines of screening and sorting patients. Many times people who stagger or dash into emergency departments are vague in describing their problems and only astute health professionals can ask the right questions and recognize impending catastrophic illnesses. Moreover, illness does not always rear its head in textbook fashion. A heart attack, for example, does not uniformly show up as chest pain: indigestion, neck, shoulder or back pain, vomiting, dizziness, arm tingling, tooth pain or just belching can be the only sign of a heart attack. Not all asthmatics wheeze and grunt heavily. The end result of these miscalculations at the initial interview can be tragic when seriously ill patients are classified as "not urgent" and sent into the waiting area. A study in the *Annals of Emergency Medicine* found that nurses, doctors and a computer program all performed poorly with triage decisions in predicting which patients actually wound up being hospitalized.[17] Ironically, patients' lives might be put at risk in the very place they came for lifesaving treatment.

Clerks, triage nurses and doctors frequently and regularly make triage errors in emergency rooms across the country. Many emergency rooms get so busy nobody is available to triage walk-in patients for minutes or hours. Alarmingly, even ill patients who arrive by ambulance frequently must wait minutes to hours to be properly evaluated and treated by a nurse and physician. The outcome of these delays can prove to be deadly.

HOW CAN I HELP HEALTHCARE PROFESSIONALS AVOID TRIAGE ERRORS?

Follow a few simple yet important rules and you will have gone a long way toward preventing your own triage travesty. Triage accuracy is in large part dependent upon how you, the patient, explain your illness or "chief complaint." For example, the man with a heart attack might have been treated more urgently if he explained that both the pain and dizziness came on suddenly and together. Patients can help healthcare professionals make quick assessments more accurate by adhering to these rules:

1. *Keep Cool*: Do not scream and flail hysterically if you are not evaluated immediately. You will be labeled histrionic or crazy and your demands for faster attention or reevaluation will not be taken seriously. Your child's cut forehead, for instance, might seem like a dire emergency to you, but to emergency staff who daily see patients on death's door, it is not a priority. Acting frightened is normal; being hysterical and unreasonable alienates those who are trying to care for you.

2. *Focus on Your Chief Complaint*: Do not reel off every ache or twitch you have had in the past month. Your credibility will fizzle as the triage nurse stops listening then interrupts you in an effort to save time and get to the point. The nurse might, in fact, cut you off before you've explained the one or two most important symptoms you've been experiencing. Mention only a few of the most recent and distressing symptoms and why they concern you now. Emergency room doctors and nurses tend to take problems less seriously when patients reel off a long list of complaints.

3. *Be Forthcoming with Relevant Information*: Tell the triage nurse:
   a. What key symptoms you are experiencing, such as difficulty breathing, headache or abdominal pain.

b.   Indicate how long these symptoms have been troubling you. Talk about one or two key associated symptoms.

c.   Mention if you have called your doctor or seen him or her in the past few days for this problem. Have you taken simple remedies such as antacids or a pain reliever or cold remedy? Having taken these medicines first and gotten no relief gives you greater credibility in triage.

d.   Know *all* medications you have recently taken or take every day including eye drops, skin creams, over-the-counter remedies, vitamins, grandma's potions and herbal elixirs. Never say, "I don't know." Carry an updated list in your wallet or purse. If necessary, just bring all your medicines in a bag when you seek medical care.

e.   Discuss any relevant past medical history. The triage nurse will approach your case differently, for instance, if she knows you had a heart attack five years ago at age thirty and you are now having chest discomfort. If you are having abdominal pain, it is important to tell the nurse if you just had a CAT scan or sonogram done a few days ago for that problem or that your appendix was removed ten years ago. Knowing when your last menstrual period was and if it has been normal and regular is vital for women of childbearing age.

f.   Carry with you your doctor's business card or name and phone number. Know with which hospital your doctor is affiliated.

g.   Voice any specific concerns to the triage nurse and doctor such as, "I'm worried it's a heart attack, because my brother died young from heart disease."

h.   If you are the stoic type and never go to doctors unless you're feeling terribly ill, by all means say so to both nurse and doctor. This is a key piece of information that would instruct any astute provider to take your complaint seriously.

4.   *Request Immediate Evaluation if Your Problem Might be Life Threatening.* If your first encounter is with a desk clerk, it is reasonable for you to request immediate evaluation by the triage nurse if you suspect your problem is potentially serious. If the triage nurse you encounter believes your problem is not serious, but you feel like it is, you can request that an emergency doctor screen you. All requests must be made in a calm and polite manner: "I'm sorry to trouble you while you're busy, but I know my son's cough is from his bad asthma."

ALARM SYMPTOMS

- Chest pain, especially if worse with exertion or a deep breath or if it travels to the back.
- Shortness of breath.
- Wheezing.
- Bleeding that does not slow or stop after placing direct pressure over the source for fifteen to thirty minutes. If blood spurts into the air, seek immediate help.
- Abdominal pain that began less than six hours ago and is severe, constant, and progressing. The pain usually prevents you from doing any routine activity.
- Loss of consciousness, feeling faint or lightheaded, limb weakness or numbness or unexplained falling.
- Heart palpitations.
- Unusually severe or worst-ever headache.
- Fever above 105 degrees.
- Persistent vomiting or severe diarrhea, particularly in infants, the elderly or those with chronic diseases like diabetes.
- When someone is exceedingly drowsy or difficult to awaken.
- Excruciating pain.
- Sudden, unexplained behavior change. Violent, paranoid, confused or self-injurious behavior.
- Severe irritability, inconsolable crying or apathy and lethargy that is unusual.
- Possible poison ingestion or drug overdose. Bring containers or bottles with you.

---

5. *Request Reevaluation if You Feel Worse.* Emergency room professionals are responsible for reevaluating all patients in the waiting area. If while you are waiting your symptoms become worse or you believe your problem has become critical, ask to be rechecked and explain why. Do not be shy. Time is of paramount importance.

6. *Help the Triage Nurse to be Thorough.* Triage booths are often not private so it can be difficult for nurses to perform a thorough screening evaluation. With breathing trouble, for instance, the nurse should listen to your chest with your shirt off, but that is often not feasible.

Unfortunately, a makeshift examination or assessment through clothing can be deceiving and dangerously lacking.

7. *Get Your Family Doctor to Meet You in the Emergency Room*: If this is
possible, a doctor who is familiar with your medical history, rather
than the emergency physician, should evaluate you. You will be
brought to an examining room as soon as your doctor arrives.
However, if your doctor is not yet there and your illness seems serious, the emergency doctor should evaluate you first.

Triage is a key aspect of emergency care, but no foolproof method
of triage exists. Much of triage is based upon the nurse's or doctor's
judgment and experience and how busy the ER is at any moment.
Never assume triage professionals must be correct in their assessments.
If your first contact is with a clerk (not a nurse or doctor) be particularly cautious and vocal if you are feeling very, and perhaps seriously, ill.
Remember that your life might depend on it!

DANGER #6
MALPRACTICE: FEARS AND FACTS

A boisterous toddler falls onto a coffee table and opens a gash on his forehead. When the emergency doctor evaluates him the boy is smiling and playful. The gash tunnels deep into the muscle layer and the hospital is wall-to-wall patients so the doctor calls the surgeon-in-training (resident) to repair the laceration.

The surgical resident briefly examines the child and asks for a suture set. As the instruments come into full view, the boy yells out, "I want to go home." The frightened boy wails and squirms as a burning novocaine injection seeps beneath his forehead skin. Two assistants restrain the child so the surgeon can stitch the wound. With each successful stitch the wound shrinks like a zipper closing. The boy has cried himself to sleep. A short while later, the surgical resident emerges from behind the curtain, removes her gloves, and fills out forms to order skull X rays.

"Why the skull films?" the emergency doctor asks.

"To rule out a fracture," she replies.

"No kidding," the emergency doctor says. "But you know very well by exam and mechanism of injury this boy has no fracture. And a child's skull films are hard to interpret..."

"Just want to be sure."

"Only sure thing about skull films is unnecessary radiation exposure," the emergency doctor insists.

"Look," the surgical resident snaps back, "some things I do for the patient and some I do for the doctor. Sutures for the child, X rays for me—for my protection." She walks away.

What this young doctor did was not illegal. Some might call her thorough in her work. Many patients would be thrilled that X rays are being ordered since a normal X ray means everything is okay, right? Wrong. The surgeon knew those films would not show her anything she didn't already know. The boy seemed fine, but if any concern did exist, it would involve an injury to the brain itself. A skull X ray shows only the skull bones, not the brain. That young surgeon was practicing "defensive" medicine.

Defensive medicine directly affects you as a patient. While it is true you do not have to write the checks each month, you are still paying for your doctor's malpractice costs and anxieties. Liability fears affect the core of medical practice. Each decision a physician makes, each test ordered, each procedure or operation performed on you, every word your doctor says (or doesn't say) to you, is tainted by fears of being sued. This directly impacts the physician-patient relationship and the medical care you receive. Malpractice fears are like a swinging axe above the heads of a physician, but many doctors have moved from their precarious positions and instead have placed patients underneath that axe.

Why do doctors perform useless tests and procedures because of fears of lawsuits? In the American medicolegal system, doing too much is safer than doing too little. Hardly a conversation passes among doctors and nurses without the poetic phrase "cover your ass" or "CYA" being voiced. An American Medical Association survey[18] of over 1000 doctors revealed that eighty-four percent of physicians perform extra tests to protect themselves from liability, resulting in over $20 billion of financial waste.[19] This figure says nothing about the risks and pain to which patients are needlessly subjected. Consider the following examples of lawsuit fears run amuck:

CASE 1

Half the physicians who staffed a small Idaho hospital emergency room resigned after a colleague lost a malpractice case.[20] That community faced inadequate physician coverage in the emergency room, the only source of emergency care in that area.

CASE 2

An internist was called to the emergency room to evaluate a young man who was experiencing chest pain. The doctor evaluated him and suspected his chest pain was not caused by a heart condition. The internist looked at the top of the computerized electrocardiogram and saw a printout of "Cannot exclude myocardial infarction." These computer readings are inaccurate and generally ignored. The electrocardiogram must be interpreted in the context of the patient's symptoms, age and heart disease risk factors.

The emergency doctor told the internist he also believed the man's symptoms were caused by intestinal problems and not a heart attack. The internist then turned to his colleague and said, "Let's admit him into the Intensive Care Unit."

"Why the ICU?" the emergency doctor asked. Another department, the "Telemetry Unit" is actually less expensive, more pleasant and beds are easier to get for heart monitoring.

The internist scratched his head. "How can I *not* send him to intensive care with 'Cannot exclude myocardial infarction' printed all over his electrocardiogram?"

In the unlikely scenario that the man *did* suffer a heart attack, the internist feared a lawsuit, because the computerized electrocardiogram "knew" the diagnosis and he ignored it. These fears might be well founded since it is easy for an attorney to say, with hindsight, how foolish a doctor was for not taking simple precautions or not making an "obvious" diagnosis that even a machine could make. In fact, about three million people are hospitalized annually for chest pain and three billion dollars are spent testing and treating those chest pain patients who, in fact, do not have serious heart disease.[21] It is up to you as a patient to protect yourself from useless and risky tests or treatments done in a defensive, medicolegal climate.

WHAT CAN YOU DO TO AVOID MALPRACTICE MANIA?

The solution to this danger is simple. Tell your doctor directly that you are interested in quality medical care, not a hefty malpractice award. Explain how you bow to common sense and compassion, not to callous or cowardly medical care. Stop the vicious cycle of liability fear leading to care that compromises a patient's best interest. End patient suspicion and mistrust of doctors; instead, do proper research to identify a competent doctor. In the emergency room setting, where you do not know your doctor, you must resort to common sense, active participation in your care and good communication. Ask appropriate questions. Do your own Web research in advance of your need for care. Be forthcoming and frank with your doctor and you will usually receive this honesty in return. For most doctors, honesty is refreshing. Common sense questions are important. Politely refuse a test if the doctor cannot logically defend the reason for exposing you to the risk or expense of it. If your doctor wants to do a blood count (CBC), for instance, ask why. Your doctor might say: "To check for signs of infection." But you are suffering from a cough and 104-degree fever. You don't need a medical degree to know you have an infection. The doctor then might say, "A low blood count suggests it might be the flu, which is treated with one type of drug, while a high blood count implies a bacterial infection which is treated with an antibiotic." That sounds logical and is worth pursuing. On the surface, it might seem terrific that your doctor thinks you are so special that you deserve spending a day or two in intensive care. If there is a well-founded concern that you have a heart problem, it is appropriate. However, when this is ordered for you and you have a negligible chance for having true heart disease based on the testing done and your medical history, you are needlessly being exposed to serious risk from infections and procedure complications. In addition, you might be subjected to an exorbitant expense for an intensive care stay, all because your doctor practices defensive medicine.

Tell your doctor you want only what is necessary to get the best care. That toddler's mother should have asked, "What is the purpose of the skull X ray?" The surgeon would have answered, "To check for a skull fracture." Mom should have inquired, "Do you strongly suspect there is a fracture?" (She might have asked the emergency doctor's opinion as well.) The surgeon's response: "Not a very high suspicion." Mom: "Is there any brain damage?" Doctor: "I doubt it." Mom: "Does the X ray show the brain?" Doctor: "No, only a CAT scan shows the brain itself." Mom: "So why get the X ray?" Doctor: "It's your child. I can't force you to have the X ray." Mom: "Thank you, but I'll pass." Doctor: "I'll simply note it on the chart that you refused the test against my advice."

If mom had pursued it further and asked for the CAT scan, the child might have undergone that test despite a normal physical examination. Be careful of what you ask for—you might get it! If it becomes necessary, inform the emergency doctor that a test will not be needed just so the doctor can "document" a normal result should a lawsuit rear its head in the future. If a doctor wants to do an arterial blood gas, for example, to check the oxygen level in your blood when you know from past experience all you need is an asthma treatment and you will be fine, tell the doctor you will pass on the additional test. Let the physician "document" in the chart that you refused the test. If this asthma attack is much more severe than usual and you are not responding to medications, perhaps the blood gas is appropriate. Make it clear that your goal is to *collaborate* with nurses and doctors in your care and to leave the emergency room on the road to healing.

RULES TO HELP NEUTRALIZE
HARMFUL EFFECTS OF DEFENSIVE MEDICINE:

- Do not request or demand tests because your neighbor or cousin once had it done. If you ask for it by name, you might end up getting the test whether or not it is medically necessary. If you question a doctor's judgment in *not* ordering a test, seek the opinion of a physician whose judgment you do trust. Do not "order" tests on your own. Do discuss all options with your doctor and inquire as to whether a certain test you read about might be useful in your case.

- Politely ask if a test, procedure or medication is truly needed. Always assume they are not needed and let the doctor or nurse provide logical reasons why they are useful. Decline a test if you do not get a logical, honest answer. If the doctor hedges or hesitates, be suspicious.
- Useful tests are those that help to "rule out" a potentially serious illness such as heart attack, appendicitis or stroke. Tests will then be useful if signs and symptoms suggest such an illness. If the doctor says, "Let's get an X ray to see what turns up," these are tests you must question, especially if they are being done so the doctor can "document" a normal result.
- Communicate with the doctor who is caring for you. Make it clear that you want only those tests or treatments that are essential. It is reasonable to allow one to three days for illness or injury to improve on its own unless the problem has real potential to threaten life or limb.
- Never say, "I'll sue you if...." when things do not go your way. ER staff will immediately avoid and isolate you. Your care will certainly suffer as a result. Doctors need some reassurance that they will be allowed to practice medicine comfortably, not fearfully. Patients can provide that reassurance and it will enhance the physician-patient relationship.

DANGER #7
PUTTING TOO MUCH TRUST IN TESTS

"I'd like an X ray just to be sure."
"Can I get a blood test so I know I'm okay?"
"There must be some test you can do to find out exactly what's wrong with me!"

Many people sanctify tests. Like primitive man's belief in magic as cause and cure for disease, modern-day patients mistakenly believe medical science offers definite answers and quick cures. Patients might feel cheated and suspicious if a doctor does not order X rays or blood tests. Consider the case of a teenage girl who bumped her head in a minor car accident. She suffered a quarter-sized lump to her forehead, but was otherwise fine. When the young lady was ready to go home from the ER, her mother balked and insisted she wanted her daughter to have a blood count and skull X rays. "I want to be sure she's not hemorrhaging and that she has no brain damage," her mother insisted. The doctor explained that bleeding into the brain cannot cause anemia, thus a blood count would prove nothing, and skull X rays do not show the brain, only skull bones. He further explained that there was no chance she had a cracked skull based on the physical examination he had performed. In the end the doctor ordered the tests to placate the teen's mother.

This case illustrates extreme patient worship of the almighty test. In truth, tests provide doctors with small clues or tidbits of information that they interpret in proper context. Tests do *not* guarantee a correct diagnosis. A "normal" test result does *not* guarantee all is okay. An "abnormal" result is *not* always a disease or problem. Indiscriminate use of tests can be dangerous for two reasons: First, a falsely abnormal result might lead patients on a path toward riskier tests and procedures. Second, test results are often "normal" in people who are truly ill, providing false reassurance that they are fine.

Are you a test worshipper? Do you believe it is always better to undergo tests or procedures to increase the chances of an accurate diagnosis? The following four categories illustrate the inaccuracy of tests—an unreliability that might turn your faith in tests into agnostic uncertainty.

IMPERFECT TESTS

A doctor confessed to his patient uncertainty about the cause for her abdominal pain. She then asked, "But didn't that blood count check for appendicitis?"

The physician explained that there is no perfect test for appendicitis. Certain tests such as blood count, sonogram and CAT scan provide clues. The patient's physical examination and symptoms also provide key information. But no single test exists which says definitely "Yes" or "No" to appendicitis. The white blood count, a measure of infection or inflammation in the body, is often elevated in those suffering from appendicitis. Many people, particularly the elderly and those in the earlier stages of appendicitis, will have a white blood count in the normal range. Tests are inherently imperfect. Even specialized CAT scans to diagnose or exclude appendicitis—the closest thing to a perfect test for this surgical emergency—can be wrong up to ten percent of the time.

Chest X rays are another example of the fallibility of tests. By the time a chest X ray shows a cancer of the lung, the disease is usually advanced. Chest X rays can help to diagnose pneumonia, yet a patient might have every sign and symptom of a lung infection and nothing will show up on the chest X ray. Moreover, pneumonia appears on X rays as white streaks in the lung amidst many "normal" white streaks. It is not always easy to tell what is normal and what is not.

Furthermore, "abnormal" results detected on an X ray or specialized test are not always true diseases. Because tests are imperfect and each person's body is unique, tests can show unexpected spots or shadows that prove to be unrelated to actual disease.

A recent and growing trend in preventive medicine is to perform a test that for years has been nothing more than the subject of medical jokes: a total body CAT scan! This is now being performed (for those who pay cash) as part of some physical examinations. Even the U.S. Army is paying for 4,000 soldiers to have it done. Sounds great except critics argue that many scans turn up some "abnormality" that might *not* be an actual disease. Such findings turn healthy people into patients who might then be subjected to risky biopsies or other procedures.[22]

Another problem that arises from inherently imperfect tests such as a total body CAT scan is when a true disease is detected (such as a tumor) long before it shows any signs or symptoms. Is that a life saved? Perhaps that tumor would never have shown signs? Perhaps that person would die of other causes long before the tumor caused any sickness? Prostate cancer, for instance, is known to be a very slow-growing tumor that is found incidentally in many older men during autopsies. Instead, the scan has transformed a healthy person into a patient who will now undergo major surgery for tumor removal or perhaps radiation therapy. These normal (or abnormal) variations among people might lead a doctor to perform risky procedures that might not have been necessary and that can lead to serious complications. The only certain thing about tests is they are uncertain and that is why there are many other components to an accurate diagnosis.

INACCURATE TESTS

Bayes' Theorem is a key scientific principle. Simply put, it states the more likely a patient is to have disease A, the more accurate will be a person's test result for disease A. Lyme disease serves as an example. If a doctor orders a Lyme test (or if a patient requests one, which happens frequently) on every person with a joint ache, fatigue or a red rash, chances go way up for a test to be falsely positive for Lyme disease. Why? Because no test is 100% perfect and other illnesses or medications can interfere with tests, rendering them inaccurate. Do you really have Lyme disease even though you live in a big city or never go in wooded areas where ticks might lurk? A positive result in such a person is likely to be falsely positive. On the other hand, negative test results often occur in those who truly have Lyme disease. The moral: Never believe a test unless the result makes sense in an individual person's situation. What's more, the current Centers for Disease Control and Prevention recommendation is *not* to order the Lyme test unless the typical rash or other symptoms are present and there is tick exposure.

A second example of Bayes' Theorem is the exercise stress test to diagnose heart disease. This commonly performed test is less accurate if done on people without major risks for heart disease. It has also been established that the exercise stress test is less accurate in women (compared with men) under age fifty. Would you believe an abnormal stress test result in a thirty-year old athlete with no risks for heart disease? That result is unlikely to be accurate. Tests do lie. Careful ordering of tests is crucial to help avoid the inaccuracies that can lead a patient on a path toward diagnostic dangers.

USELESS TESTS

Some doctors order useless tests. I define a "useless test" as one providing no new and important information or providing information that in no way changes the plan of treatment or long term outlook. Skull X rays fit into this category. Numerous studies have concluded that skull X rays provide little useful information, are difficult to interpret, tell nothing about the brain itself and can contribute to cataract formation in children. Few good reasons remain for ordering a skull X ray since the widespread availability of the CAT scan, yet these films are still ordered routinely. The CAT scan, in fact, does show the brain itself and detects skull fractures more accurately than skull X rays.

As another example of useless tests, primary care or emergency doctors might order a blood count (CBC) in infants over six months of age or young children with a fever of 104 degrees. If the child is active and has an infected throat or ear, for instance, this test is rarely useful and causes needless discomfort. An elevated white blood count is expected in such a child and should not be alarming. Treatment for an active child with an identifiable source of infection is unlikely to change based on that blood test.

Lower back X rays are yet another example of a frequently useless test. Many studies have found that plain back X rays provide little useful information when done on patients who simply wrench their back and suffer muscular strains without a serious fall or accident. Yet a large number of patients who twist their back will get these spine X rays in an emergency room or urgent care facility, needlessly subjecting them to a hefty dose of radiation.

MISINTERPRETED TESTS

Tests are imperfect and inaccurate and those who interpret them sometimes err as well. Most emergency room doctors have no expert training in interpreting X rays, CAT scans or MRIs and they commonly misread these tests. What's more, emergency room doctors at community hospitals might be forced to interpret a brain CAT scan, for instance, when a radiologist is not available after office hours. The consequences can be disastrous since brain bleeds or strokes are commonly missed diagnoses. A study published in a respected medical journal found that emergency room doctors misinterpreted a brain CAT scan in over one third of 555 cases.[23] Nearly two-thirds of these errant readings by emergency doctors had the potential for serious consequences to the patient, according to the study. Alarmingly, radiologists also frequently misinterpret X rays, CAT scans and other radiology tests despite being the experts.

Electrocardiograms that are done to check for heart disease or heart attack frequently are misinterpreted as well. Incredibly, as many as one in twenty people suffering a heart attack who complain of chest pain are mistakenly sent home from emergency rooms.

Doctors misinterpret blood tests, too. A normal white blood count might be reassuring to an inexperienced doctor, but it is no guarantee someone with abdominal pain does not have appendicitis or another serious problem. This is particularly true in infants and the elderly.

The lesson to be learned: When a doctor tells you your test result was "okay," it does not guarantee you have no serious medical problem. A corollary to that rule: Ordering a few tests does not guarantee your doctor will come up with a definite or accurate diagnosis. It is abundantly clear tests can give false reassurance or lead to needless worry and riskier tests or procedures. Another consideration is that each test ordered will prolong your emergency room stay. Radiology and laboratory tests can increase the time you spend in the emergency room by several hours. With emergency rooms already overburdened, the longer wait you experience from testing backup adds to patient frustration and emergency department confusion. You might accept a longer wait believing additional tests will provide definite or important answers, but imagine your frustration once you know how uncertain and useless some of these tests can be.

ELIMINATING TEST WORSHIP

Trust tests only if they make sense in the context of your symptoms, examination and medical history, otherwise avoid them when possible.

An important part of common sense is to ask the proper questions before agreeing to any test. For instance:

- What is the name of the test?
- What can it show? How helpful will it be in my case?
- How accurate is the test? Can it give misleading information? Doctors might use the terms false positive and false negative rates to answer these questions. False positive means the test says you have a problem when you really do not. False negative means the test says you do *not* have the disease when, in fact, you *do* suffer from it.
- How experienced is the person who is performing the test or procedure? A sonogram is only as good as the technician who performs the test and the quality of the sonogram machine. If the technician does not get the needed views and angles, the diagnosis will be missed. Similarly, mammograms must be interpreted by experts and must be of sufficient quality for these X rays to be useful in properly diagnosing breast cancer. When an unskilled or inexperienced doctor performs a biopsy, if the needed cells or tissues are missed, the diagnosis will be missed, too.

- Will the test result change the plan of treatment? If you treat both a broken toe and a bruised toe by wrapping it with tape, why X ray a stubbed toe?
- How safe is the test? What is the most common complication or danger? What is the most serious risk? Are there safer alternatives?
- How much does the test cost? Will my insurance pay for the test?

Accept the inescapable fact that tests and procedures have serious limitations. Both patients and doctors would like to believe they have all the answers with a simple test, but it just is not true. Tests are uncertain and the sooner you accept this fact, the sooner you will become a safer and more savvy patient.

X RAY CAVEATS: TIPS TO AVOID CONFUSION

If you agree to get an X ray, beware of trigger-happy doctors, nurses and technologists. You might have a bruise under your left eye, for example, but an entire facial series will be done automatically, including jaws and cheekbones far removed from your injury. Why not get an isolated X ray for an isolated injury regardless of what a radiologist who is not present might want? Two or three views of the same injured area, on the other hand, can be helpful in spotting a subtle fracture or clarifying the extent of an obvious one. Clarify with doctor and technologist exactly how many X rays truly need to be taken, the site of your injury and where the point of maximal pain is located.

Children are often subjected to "comparison" views of an uninjured limb to check for subtle fractures, especially for growth plate injuries. A growth plate injury sounds terrible, but most of these injuries are minor and will not affect growth. Never allow these comparison views to be done until after the doctor evaluates the X ray of the injured side. If the doctor has serious concerns that might alter treatment then it is reasonable to get comparison views of the good side.

Another caveat: X rays are mistakenly done on the wrong side of the body as often as three-year-olds put the left shoe on the right foot. Be alert and clarify right versus left side, the number of X rays that are actually needed (as opposed to "It's part of a series so the radiologist will want all the views") and the precise location of maximal pain or where the problem is. Communicate with doctor and technician and politely refuse useless views.

Never allow an X-ray technician to needlessly expand the field of radiation exposure because of his or her laziness or ineptitude. A spine X ray on a child with scoliosis, for instance, should be focused onto one small sheet of X-ray film. It should not be done using a long, folded film that also radiates the child's pelvis and head. The field must be as focused as possible to limit body exposure to radiation. This is particularly important for sensitive areas in a growing child (or adult) including the reproductive organs, thyroid gland, breasts, eyes and brain. Appropriate shields should be used whenever possible.

DANGER #8
DON'T WEAR THE "SERVICE PATIENT" LABEL

"Service patient" is a label that carries no prestige. Millions of people on welfare or without medical insurance know this too well. What exactly is a "service patient?" A person who needs hospital admission or emergency department specialist care, but who has welfare insurance or no insurance at all, will be branded a "service patient." That means the on-call doctor (via a predetermined schedule) will be called in to take responsibility for the individual's medical care. At teaching hospitals, inexperienced doctors-in-training will manage the care for service patients. Do you have medical insurance? Even if the answer is "yes," do not yet exhale a sigh of relief. If you end up needing care at an unfamiliar hospital where your family doctor does not have privileges, you too might be branded a "service patient." At that unfamiliar hospital, if you require specialist care or hospital admission, most doctors would rather not come to the hospital after office hours or overnight. Emergency staff would then notify the on-call specialist to take your case, offering a hit or miss approach to your medical crisis.

DO "SERVICE PATIENTS" RECEIVE SUB-PAR MEDICAL CARE?

Everyone in this country has a right to receive medical care, but free care does not guarantee quality care. There appears to be two levels of medical care—better quality care for the insured, second-rate care for those who cannot pay. The number of people who are uninsured is rising as insurance premiums become unaffordable for individuals and employers. Sadly, about forty-four million people are now in the second-class tier of care.

A recent study from the National Institutes of Health in Bethesda, Maryland found that people who had Medicaid welfare insurance or no health insurance had higher overall death rates than those with employer-provided insurance. A Harvard Medical School study found that uninsured patients were twice as likely to receive substandard care than people who were insured.[24] *The Journal of the American Medical Association* reported that the uninsured or those with welfare insurance were more frequently hospitalized for illnesses that could have been treated without hospitalization.[25] Other studies have shown that those who are uninsured are more likely to suffer delays in receiving care, are less likely to get preventive services and are treated differently than those with health insurance while in the hospital.[26]

Furthermore, follow-up care at hospital clinics is limited and slipshod at best since appointments are filled for weeks to months in advance. Doctors' offices frequently do not see patients with welfare insurance since reimbursement barely covers paperwork expenses. Thus medical care for "service patients" becomes fragmented. Those who suffer from chronic illness like diabetes develop complications because of poor medical management. They then wind up sicker and back in the emergency room.

Care for "service patients" in the emergency department and hospital do not fare any better. Chaotic emergency departments are fertile ground for negligent care, according to The Harvard Medical Practice Study II.[27] Who cares for these patients in the hospital or emergency room setting? Inexperienced doctors-in-training are primarily responsible for the care of "service patients." When experienced specialists are called to treat these patients, they often refuse or try to pass the burden on to other doctors.

How can you, a hard-working and insured person, wind up in a Russian roulette game with your healthcare? If you are traveling away from home and become ill, you will be taken to a hospital where your physician undoubtedly does not have admitting privileges. In unfamiliar territory, you too might be classified as a "service patient."

There are several dangers to wearing the "service patient" label. If you need care from a specialist, emergency staff will call the doctor "on the board" based on a predetermined call schedule. The on-call specialist who treats you might be totally incompetent, an expert in the field or somewhere in between. It's a toss up, a roll of the dice, a spin of the wheel. The quality of the doctor who will operate on you or treat your heart attack or set your broken bone is unpredictable. Even the most prestigious hospitals have poorly skilled physicians on staff. At a teaching hospital, the physician who treats "service patients" will most likely be an inexperienced doctor-in-training (Resident) who gets little guidance from more experienced physicians. A second danger is that most on-call specialists do not want to be bothered with "service patients."

"Service patients" are an extra burden to physicians with hectic schedules and there is a good chance they will not get paid much, if anything. It is disheartening that one of the first questions some specialists ask the emergency physician is, "Does the patient have insurance?" Treatment is quite different when the patient has no insurance (if the specialist will even agree to treat an uninsured patient) as opposed to the treatment given an insured individual. For example, those with no insurance (or welfare) are less likely to get a cast applied promptly for a fracture. The uninsured patient will be sent to an orthopedic clinic for follow-up care in several days. At community hospitals, the orthopedist, rather than rushing to the hospital when called for the patient, might meet uninsured patients in the emergency department the following day, which is a great inconvenience to someone who is in pain and hobbling around on crutches.

A third danger of the "service patient" label is that the "lazy admission" will more likely be used for patients who need or perhaps don't need hospital admission. I define "lazy admission" as an unnecessary hospital admission for the doctor's convenience or appropriately admitting a patient into the hospital, but neglecting traditional human physician responsibilities. This means the admitting doctor will not promptly evaluate the individual in the emergency room to double-check the plan of care set by the ER doctor. "Service patients" often get no explanations, no reassurance and no handholding. Daily hospital visits from the admitting doctor might be fleeting. The physician also has every incentive to discharge "service patients" early to eliminate another burden from his or her duties.

PEELING OFF THE "SERVICE PATIENT" LABEL

Never allow this label to stick. To allow that is to risk shoddy medical care. How can you avoid the sticky "service patient" label? Here are some ways to protect yourself:

1. The surest way to avoid this dilemma is to seek emergency care at a hospital at which your family doctor has admitting privileges (assuming you have established a good relationship with a reliable primary care physician). Any emergency care you require can then be done under guidance from your family doctor.
2. Should unexpected illness land you in an unfamiliar hospital, contact your family doctor. He or she might know a quality physician to recommend at that unfamiliar hospital.
3. It is a good idea to learn in advance the name of a competent internist or pediatrician at nearby hospitals, particularly a university hospital. You might one day need specialized trauma, heart or pediatric intensive care services. Contacting that doctor yourself or having your family doctor make the call can streamline care during that type of emergency.

4. Communicate and ask questions if you wind up at an unfamiliar hospital emergency room or if you have no family doctor. Do not passively allow emergency staff to decide who will be your admitting physician or treating specialist (if you require either). Do not allow inexperienced doctors-in-training or shoddy specialists to manage your care. You should make every effort to bypass the on-call list of unpredictable specialists by "requesting" a doctor by name.

5. Ask questions. Speak with nurses, emergency doctors or training physicians and find out who is skilled in a particular field. You will likely get truthful answers or a telling facial gesture if you are polite and persistent.

6. At the very least, demand that a Senior or Chief Resident oversee or provide your treatment.

DANGER #9
LOSING THE CRUCIAL
"GOLDEN HOUR" OF TREATMENT

The "Golden Hour" is that crucial sixty-minute period immediately following the onset of a serious injury (or illness). To get optimum care within this time period, the patient must be rushed to a hospital to be stabilized, then undergo emergency surgery or a lifesaving procedure. Each minute of delay reduces chances for survival. What you might not know is that chances for survival from severe injury or illness depends in large part upon the hospital to which you are taken.

A woman crashes her car into a pole. A man experiences crushing chest pain. While climbing a tree, a child falls and strikes his head on the ground. Should these seriously ill or injured people be rushed to the nearest hospital? Not necessarily. As one emergency department director once said, "Surviving certain life-threatening emergencies is a matter of being in the right place at the right time."

Under dire medical circumstances, your life will depend upon two key factors. The common denominators for success in treating catastrophic injury or illness are prompt care by skilled physicians and the availability of hi-tech resources.

PHYSICIAN SKILL

Trauma centers are usually large teaching hospitals that have trauma teams of surgeons who can get to the emergency room any hour of the day within one or two minutes. Many of the doctors on trauma teams are still in training, but the team does have experienced doctors with expertise in treating limb-or life-threatening injuries. By contrast, an emergency room physician working at a community hospital treats just a few seriously injured patients in a year compared with hundreds or thousands treated at trauma centers. *The more you do something, the better you do it*. This is a key concept to bear in mind when getting specialized medical care or procedure-oriented treatments such as:
- Major and complex surgery
- Heart angiogram or other invasive cardiac procedure
- Trauma care for a serious injury or burn
- Pediatric critical care
- Specialized medical care for obscure or difficult to treat disease

The more you do something, the better you get at it. It's a simple principle that makes sense and studies have confirmed this intuitive concept. A recent report in the respected *Journal of the American Medical Association* confirmed previous studies that have shown lower death rates for high-risk procedures that are performed at hospitals with a high volume of that procedure.[28] The lower death rates likely reflect more skilled surgeons, fewer technical errors with the procedure and more skilled anesthesia and postoperative care.[29]

Are you more likely to receive better care for a seriously ill or injured child at a community hospital or teaching hospital emergency room? The community hospital is staffed by doctors and nurses who have little experience treating seriously ill babies and young children; teaching hospitals, by contrast, might have separate pediatric emergency areas staffed only by pediatricians who are experts in caring for children and babies. Any hospital that has a pediatric intensive care unit on site will likely be better prepared and able to treat your child's serious illness or injury.

The same principles apply for breathing and heart emergencies. If the emergency room doctor has difficulty placing a breathing tube for respiratory failure or inserting a pacemaker to jump-start a stalled heart, an expert in those respective fields can take charge within two minutes at a teaching hospital. In many community hospitals, help might not arrive for many minutes in life or death crises—help that may be too little, too late.

Simply put, the quality of your medical care at community hospitals is highly dependent on the skills of the emergency room physician. Few if any specialists are immediately available at community hospitals, particularly during late night or early morning hours. Even getting commonplace tests such as an emergency CAT scan at a quality community hospital might be delayed minutes to hours, because the technician must be called in from home. As precious minutes pass, the "golden hour" is quickly becoming time-tarnished.

In keeping with the key concept of the "golden hour," trauma centers have specialists from all fields in the hospital twenty-four hours every day. The injured patient can be in the operating room getting lifesaving treatment within minutes. Numerous studies have confirmed that death and disability rates are lowered when seriously injured patients are taken directly to a trauma center. Care can be good at a quality community hospital, but patients will have a better chance for recovery with immediately available specialist care and prompt performance of lifesaving procedures. University hospitals do more high risk and specialized tests and procedures. In addition, when specialists must be called in from home as at community and rural hospitals, precious time is wasted. A person who suffers severe brain injury, for instance, might have a chance to survive if a neurosurgeon can operate within minutes to release blood clots in the brain. Most community hospitals cannot offer instantaneous care by a skilled neurosurgeon.

It is also troubling that many community hospital emergency room workers consider major trauma or illness as a stressful event that will tie up the one or two doctors and few nurses, slowing emergency department flow. Trauma centers call a trauma team of surgeons who are prepared to treat major injuries; cardiology Fellows at teaching hospitals eagerly await the arrival of critically ill heart patients to decide if they require emergency procedures such as angioplasty or a pacemaker.

When specialists with expertise and experience are immediately available to care for your serious illness or injury, it can make the difference between life and death.

AVAILABILITY OF SPECIALIZED RESOURCES

Another major consideration in choosing a hospital for emergency care is knowing which hospitals offer the latest lifesaving technologies. Community hospitals usually do not perform open-heart surgery or emergency balloon angioplasty (opening of clogged heart arteries) during a massive heart attack. A device called an intra-aortic balloon pump can keep alive certain patients who are suffering from a massive heart attack or severe angina. This, too, is unavailable at most community hospitals. At smaller hospitals, the resources and expense required to provide these services are prohibitive.

Clearly, differences exist among hospitals and their emergency rooms. Your chances for survival from serious illness or injury are greater at a university hospital with high-level trauma care. Being in the right place at the right time can truly save your life.

HOW TO AVOID POORLY EQUIPPED FACILITIES

It is your task as an informed and prepared health consumer to find out about the hospitals in your community. Do this *now*, not en route to the emergency room in a cloud of panic. How can you find out which hospitals offer expert care in various fields? You have several resources at your disposal.
1. Ask your family doctor which nearby hospital is a high-level trauma and teaching hospital. Better yet, use as your primary care physician

a doctor who is affiliated with a trauma or teaching hospital. Should you need specialized emergency care, an extra few minutes in the ambulance is worthwhile to get to the best-equipped hospital.

2. Call the Public Relations Department of all nearby hospitals and have them send you brochures that promote the hospital's areas of expertise. Ask them if they offer specialty care in areas such as:

- Level One trauma care, including helicopter transport of critically ill or injured people for rapid treatment during the "Golden Hour"
- Invasive heart care including emergency balloon angioplasty and heart bypass surgery (twenty-four hours daily)
- Pediatric intensive care
- High-risk obstetrics
- Neonatal intensive care
- Special emergency department care such as a separate heart evaluation unit for rapid diagnosis and treatment of heart attacks; a separate pediatric emergency division staffed by pediatricians; a separate psychiatric emergency area.
- Cancer care including the latest experimental treatments
- Burn unit
- Medical school affiliation

3. Ask friends and relatives who had excellent care at a hospital to give you a recommendation.

4. A trip to the library or a Web search can provide a treasure trove of information. Magazines and newspapers frequently do special reports on medical care at regional hospitals or emergency rooms. *U.S. News and World Report*, for instance, rates the best hospitals nationwide. Many regional magazines and newspapers rate "the best" doctors. Needless to say these ratings must be considered with some skepticism, but they can offer guidance. Many hospitals now have their own Web sites that include much of the above information. Call your local or state Health Department (or log on to their Web site). Some states are now required to release a hospital "report card" to the public. The report card includes patient death or bad outcome rates in many specialties and various surgical procedures (search "Hospital Report Card" or "Hospital Mortality" or "Hospital Morbidity" on the Web). Note: Proponents are quick to point out that death rates for open-heart surgery have dropped by fifty percent since individual New York hospital death rates were made available to the public in 1989. Critics claim many hospitals will now turn away the sickest patients

since death rates are likely to go higher when treating extremely ill patients. Similarly, hospitals that treat the sickest patients might have higher death rates because no other facility would risk caring for those sick patients. Find out if your State Health Department releases this information and use it, but know its inherent limitations.

Some states, including Massachusetts and Florida, have made individual doctor profiles available through databases accessible to the public. The World Wide Web offers many sites that provide hospital and doctor information. Available sites include those from individual hospitals, medical organizations such as the American Medical Association doctor and hospital finders, local and state health departments or online magazines such as US News Online.

5. Get a Medic Alert Bracelet. This will help to ensure that you are taken to the appropriate hospital or emergency department in a crisis situation, particularly if you have special medical needs. This bracelet can list your special medical problems, drug allergies, doctor and hospital at which you receive care.

6. Communicate with the ambulance crew that will transport you to a hospital. If your condition is immediately life threatening, they might have to take you to the nearest emergency room. If your condition is stable, the crew can transport you to the hospital of your choice within that community. For serious injury, pediatric illness or heart problems that are not imminently life threatening, the ambulance crew should take you to the appropriate hospital in the area that offers expert treatment.

7. Map out the quickest route to each hospital on your list in case of illness or injury that is not serious enough to warrant ambulance transport.

USEFUL WEB SITES

http://www.bestdoctors.com
(This referral service helps patients find the best doctors and hospitals for their needs.)

http://thriveonline.oxygen.com/medical/powerful/besthospital.html
(This site holds healthcare information in the article, "Find the Best Hospital" as well as links to various hospital directories.)

http://www.castleconnolly.com
(This site is a guide to help healthcare consumers find excellent physicians in every hospital in the United States and beyond.)

DANGER #10
YOUR LAST REQUESTS CAN BE IGNORED

Mary stared at the ceiling in the intensive care unit, disturbed by beeping monitors and droning machines. Only those plastic tubes stuffed down her throat could stop her from yelling loudly. Mary's spunk and free-spirited nature had not waned even after eighty years. She ignored doctors who for forty years admonished her to stop her two vices: smoking and drinking. Mary outlived them all. That day, she arrived at the emergency room gasping for air. Her lips were blue, skin ashen, flabby muscles fatigued and heart weary. Emphysema had caught up with Mary. She grimaced and waved the doctor away, but was too winded to speak her mind. The emergency room doctor had seen many "combative" patients suffering from air hunger. Mary's arms flailed trying to stop the inevitable. The doctor ignored her gestures and administered an intravenous sedative. A soporific haze quieted Mary's protests while the doctor inserted a breathing tube into her windpipe then connected the tube to a respirator.

Mary's lungs filled with air like inflating party balloons. Silently, she told herself she could never forgive the emergency room doctor for saving her life. Mary was angry with the ER doctor for saving her life, because she had signed Do Not Resuscitate (DNR) forms. Mary had decided long ago that she wanted to die gracefully—the way she had lived. She would not be kept alive by noisy respirators. She would have no part of those intensive care units where she would not be permitted to smoke or drink. Mary never allowed anyone to tell her what to do during her life. "Sure won't let doctors and nurses pound on my chest when I die," she once said. With a chuckle she added, "The day I die is the one day in my life I'd like to have some peace and quiet."

Mary had signed DNR papers that legally bound physicians to honor her wishes not to receive extraordinary treatments such as chest compressions or being hooked up to a respirator. Sadly, it is common for patients like Mary to arrive at an emergency room alone, unable to speak and without the paperwork that documents those wishes. The emergency physician and paramedics are then legally obligated to do everything to save that patient's life. Fearing law suits, many emergency physicians will knowingly disobey such a wish, even if the patient is able to vocalize it, if adequate legal documentation is not in hand. Mary had to suffer for three weeks with tubes down her throat and dozens of needle sticks until she finally died. Mary celebrated life, but her final days were no party.

ADVANCE DIRECTIVES 101

A Healthcare Advance Directive is a legal document or contract giving healthcare workers instructions for making decisions in your care if you cannot communicate your wishes. Needless to say, a directive is meaningless unless doctors and nurses know about and see it. Advance Directives are not just for the seriously or terminally ill. Everyone should prepare one in case tragedy strikes. Advance directives enable you to give specific instructions about treatments you *do* or do not want when terminally ill or comatose. They also apply for any temporary or permanent impairment.

Why go through the unpleasant task of preparing an Advance Directive? This document will enable your family and treating doctor to know your true wishes regarding extraordinary medical treatments and life prolongation. Another key benefit of a directive is that it will remove the burdens of making life and death decisions from family members. Do not underestimate the emotional turmoil and guilt felt by a family member who must allow a loved one to die naturally, knowing there are extraordinary measures that might keep the person alive. Family members often believe they are "killing" the loved one by withholding treatment and letting them go. What's more, when family members are left to decide about life support decisions, philosophical disagreement among family members is common, leading to estrangements during an already difficult time.

There are a few options available for Healthcare Advance Directives, usually requiring special forms, signing procedures and witnesses. Each state has its own particular regulations. The good news is that recent legislation in many states has made it easier and more reliable to have "do not resuscitate" wishes honored by doctors and paramedics during a crisis. Another advantage to preparing an Advance Directive: not only can you name an individual to act as your "Agent" to enforce your wishes, but you can even name those people you want *excluded* from making any decision on your behalf. Be sure that any person you appoint as your "Proxy" or "Agent" has similar philosophies about life and death and a clear understanding of your wishes.

Three commonly used Advance Directives are Healthcare Directive (Living Will), Healthcare Proxy and Do Not Resuscitate (DNR) forms.

Healthcare Directive (Living Will, Directive to Physicians)

This is a written instruction detailing your wishes to include or exclude specific types of medical treatment whether permanently or temporarily impaired or terminally ill. Some key aspects to the Living Will include:

- The ability to name an Agent and Alternate Agent to make decisions for your medical care if you cannot. The Living Will can limit in any way the decision-making power of the Agent and can include organ donation wishes.

- A Living Will should state specific goals for treatment and care, such as your wish not to live without meaningful higher brain function or whether you would not want to live on a ventilator or with loss of mobility.
- A Living Will may include a values history, which discusses the subject's personal feelings about life and death, pain and suffering, religious values, children, past experiences and how these play in the decision to live or die.

Healthcare Proxy (Healthcare Durable Power of Attorney)

Another directive option is the Healthcare Proxy or Durable Power of Attorney. This document gives a named individual authority to make medical care decisions for you, without specifying what treatments you would want. For this reason, the Proxy should be done in combination with a Living Will so the Agent you choose can help to honor your wishes specified in the Living Will.

Do Not Resuscitate (DNR)

This form instructs healthcare workers not to perform cardiopulmonary resuscitation (CPR) or hook you up to a respirator if your heart stops or if you stop breathing. Family members or a designated Agent can implement a DNR on your behalf after doctors declare you terminally ill and unable to participate in this decision.

A major dilemma has always been that a DNR status is only useful if healthcare workers know about it, as Mary's experience illustrates. Moreover, even if paramedics or doctors knew about the patient's wishes, they would not honor them unless legal documentation was in hand, because of fears of being sued. Many states now recognize DNR bracelets that are worn around the wrist or ankle so paramedics and doctors immediately know they can legally honor a patient's wish to die naturally without intervention. The bracelets can only be obtained through a specific process and agency which varies by state. States that recognize DNR bracelets are: New York, Connecticut, Wisconsin, Massachusetts, California, Indiana, Kansas, Maryland, Louisiana, Nevada and New Mexico.

AVOIDING MARY'S SUFFERING AND LOSS OF DIGNITY

It isn't simple to do, but don't get angry like Mary did—get ready. Plan ahead. If you are twenty-eight and healthy, now is the perfect time to write in a living will your wishes should you forget to replace your worn car brakes. "I am of sound mind and feel strongly that I want everything done to save me due to religious beliefs." Or if you prefer, "I am of sound mind. I watched my father suffer a long and painful death and I'm sure it's not for me. If there is no hope for a meaningful life with higher brain function, give my organs to someone who needs them." If you are seriously ill: "I am of sound mind....I suffer from excruciating pain everyday and do not want a tube placed in my throat nor chest compressions (CPR) performed should my heart or breathing stop. If I am permanently unconscious, I do not want a feeding tube placed in me to prolong my suffering." Many states have implemented proxy laws which allow a patient to give decision-making powers to a trusted person (a surrogate) if the patient is unable to make his or her own decisions. A reminder: Be certain that the surrogate you choose understands your wishes and has a similar philosophy about suffering and life prolongation. Misunderstandings can lead to indecision during a time of crisis.

Important Tips To Improve Chances Your Advance Directive Will Be Enforced

- Choose a Proxy or Agent you trust to help honor your wishes. This person would best serve your needs if he or she is assertive, willing to spend time by your side at the hospital and someone who lives locally.
- Give a copy of your Advance Directive to your doctor, Healthcare Agent, hospital, and/or nursing home.
- Discuss your wishes and values in detail with both your doctor and designated Agent.
- Keep in your wallet or purse a card indicating you have an Advance Directive.
- Let family members and your attorney know where you keep it.
- For those who are seriously ill, terminally ill or elderly, once you've made a Do Not Resuscitate decision, there are several ways to improve your chances it will be enforced. Send a copy of your DNR paperwork to all local emergency rooms and request that a copy be distributed to all emergency doctors and nurses at those hospitals. Do the same with paramedics in your community since paramedics might unknowingly place a breathing tube into your throat before you arrive at the emergency room. DNR bracelets or a Medic Alert bracelet indicating your DNR status are other approaches. One option rarely used in this country for the terminally ill is to tell family members or neighbors *not* to call an ambulance when the

final event strikes. Allow the terminally ill person to die peacefully at home. This is, however, understandably a difficult decision for loved ones.

- For more information on these important issues and state-by-state information about Advance Directives contact:
  1. Your State Health Department
  2. Choice In Dying, Inc.: 1-800-989-WILL
  3. Legal Counsel for the Elderly: 202-434-2120
  4. Your Hospital Patient Representative or Advocate
  5. Administration on Aging: 202-619-7501

USEFUL WEB SITES

http://www.aarp.org

(The Web site of the American Association of Retired Persons, a non-profit member organization for people ages 50 and over.)

http://www.aoa.gov

(The Administration on Aging offers services and information for older Americans and their families to create opportunities for and meet the needs of older persons at risk of losing their independence.)

http://www.nolo.com

(Nolo offers legal information online and publishes self-help legal books, forms and software in plain, readable English for the general public.)

http://www.choices.org

(Choice In Dying, Inc., the inventors of living wills in 1967, is dedicated to aiding individuals in making end-of-life decisions.)

DANGER #11
"LAZY ADMISSIONS"
AND OTHER ADMITTING ATROCITIES

An overnight stay in the hospital is no night at a four-star hotel: bare white walls, moaning patients and rank odors wafting across hallways. Roommates have a habit of watching late-night television on high volume. Nurses will awaken you frequently during the night for routine checks. These are just a few of the apparent problems. Hazards you cannot see include resistant infections spread among patients by healthcare workers as well as needle sticks, tests and treatments that pose dangers.

Getting admitted into a hospital is a traumatic experience. Many questions flash through your head. Who will care for the children? What will I do about that foot-high stack of papers on my office desk? Is my illness serious? Will I suffer permanent disability? How do I know these doctors are on the right track? Are they doing everything necessary to diagnose and treat my illness with minimal pain and risk to me? Who will feed the dog or cat? Will I be able to pay the mortgage at the end of the month? Will insurance cover this? Am I going to die?

Before your harried brain can come up with answers to these questions, you get pinched, poked and prodded like a pincushion. Blood tests, IVs and other prickly procedures await you. In your state of panic, there are three things you need most: A strong dose of reassurance from an individual you trust; explanations about the working diagnosis and all test and treatment options; a solid game plan for pain relief and illness treatment while avoiding needless harm or injury.

Who can supply all these wonders? You won't need a guardian angel or a fairy godmother. A dedicated and competent private (family) doctor should be able to provide the reassurance and treatment you deserve. The first day illness or injury strikes is the most traumatic. Without warning, you are hurled into the role of patient. The disease might be progressing or may still be undiagnosed. You are in severe pain or perhaps vomiting or turning yellow. Now would be a great time for a little handholding and calming words. Simple explanations from a concerned expert who is planning your care would be reassuring. The emergency room doctor, unfortunately, cannot give each patient the time needed to live up to these expectations.

Many primary care (family) doctors *do* live up to these responsibilities, but others rely on the "lazy admission." As I defined it earlier, a "lazy admission" is an unnecessary hospital admission for the doctor's convenience or appropriately admitting a patient into the hospital, but neglecting one or all of the three key physician responsibilities.

DUBIOUS ADMISSIONS

Why would a doctor unnecessarily admit a patient into the hospital? There are many possible explanations, but the most common are familiar to you: fear, greed and laziness. Fear of malpractice liability for a bad outcome; financial gain for procedures and daily hospital visit reimbursements; and laziness, because it is easier to admit a patient with multiple medical problems than to go to the hospital ER, sort through his or her chart and many problems to determine what is new and what is baseline, provide needed reassurance and treatment, then send the patient home.

Fear of being sued is a powerful motivator for needless hospital admissions. It is most evident with patients experiencing chest pain. A twinge of chest pain might land a patient in the hospital. The majority of these patients wind up not having a heart problem or heart attack. This "better safe than sorry" approach causes many people to be admitted into the hospital when only a few truly need it. Common sense, careful evaluation and close follow-up could help to avoid many needless admissions.

Another reason some physicians admit patients is for financial gain. Doctors can bill insurance companies for daily hospital visits even if that visit lasts only sixty seconds (some physicians might not show up at all on several days). The hospitalization also gives a greedy doctor an opportunity to perform unnecessary procedures such as heart catheterization, surgery or colonoscopy. Perhaps more importantly, when a physician admits many patients into the hospital, that doctor keeps hospital business booming, leading to greater hospital revenues. This physician might be rewarded with various incentives like getting "unavailable" beds for patients when needed, having more clout in hospital decision-making politics or even titles and promotions. Former Surgeon-General C. Everett Koop, in his Ten-point Proposal for Revitalizing Primary Care, cites a study showing that hospital care in Boston costs twice as much per capita as in New Haven, Connecticut, yet patient death is similar in both cities. He explains that the disparity exists because Boston has more hospital beds available, "and where beds exist, they will be filled," Koop says in the proposal. A large subgroup of patients who are admitted into the hospital can get equally good care without the hospital stay.

The third reason for needless admissions is laziness. It is easier to admit a patient over the telephone instead of making a trip to the emergency department, doing a thorough evaluation and possibly sending the patient home with close follow-up care. Even if admission is necessary, doctors often will not come in to see the patient until the next morning. I call these admissions "lazy admissions," because the patient is cheated out of needed reassurance and more thorough care.

When a family doctor does not promptly evaluate a patient at the hospital, three possible admitting scenarios exist. At teaching hospitals, an inexperienced medical student, intern or second-year training doctor will oversee the immediate plan of care and write orders for admission and preliminary tests. This might be done with minimal guidance from the patient's more experienced private doctor. At community hospitals, it is common for private doctors to give a nurse verbal orders (over the telephone) for medications and necessary tests. This is often done at 3:00 A.M. while the doctor is still yawning in bed. All these critical decisions are made weary-eyed and without the patient's doctor performing an examination! Doctors responsible for admitting a patient frequently do not even speak with the emergency doctor who *did* examine their patient. Another possible scenario is the hurried emergency doctor scribbling a few orders to get the patient admitted. Lazy admissions occur most commonly with patients who are unfamiliar to the admitting doctor, patients without insurance and when one doctor is covering another doctor's patients for a night, weekend or during vacation. But the "lazy admission" can victimize anyone if a family physician or specialist who is admitting someone into the hospital does not promptly evaluate his or her patient.

But what is the harm in playing it safe and keeping a patient in the hospital? Charles' story will help to explain. Charles had a "baggy" heart and suffered from bouts of water in his lungs. An occasional dietary indiscretion or worsening heart function would tip him into heart failure. This time his doctor decided to treat him in the hospital with intravenous medication rather than extra water pills at home. "Just a two-day tune up," his doctor joked.

Two days later, Charles developed shaking chills and a fever of 104 degrees. Charles had developed a full-blown infection and clotting of the vein at the intravenous site—a complication called thrombophlebitis. He would now require potent antibiotics during a six-week hospital stay. The next day Charles was taken to the operating room to have that vein removed for fear the infection would not clear. A two-day "tune up" turned into a life-threatening ordeal for Charles. Similar hospital-related complications occur everyday in our country's institutions of healing.

Older People at Risk

The elderly are at particularly high risk for bad outcomes from avoidable hospitalizations, tests or procedures since they have less reserves of kidney and liver function, frequently suffer from multiple medical problems, often take many medications and may be in delicate health. Avoidable and "lazy admissions" commonly occur with frail, elderly or nursing home patients, people who, as a group, are most susceptible to hospital or doctor induced complications (called iatrogenic illness).

Complications of hospitalization and medical treatment occur more commonly in the elderly and can be more severe. Injuries resulting from medical care (iatrogenic) include serious hospital-acquired infections like pneumonia, bad reactions to drugs, falls, bedsores, complications of surgery or other procedures and mental confusion from the stress of hospitalization. Because the elderly have less reserves in body function, they are at great risk for cascade iatrogenesis, a domino effect of one complication following another, which is common in people with limited reserves for coping with mental and physical stress.

Other factors contributing to an increased vulnerability of the elderly in hospital settings include greater passivity by elderly patients, a tendency to give vague medical histories and healthcare providers attributing symptoms of illness to "old age." Less typical manifestations of serious illness can also delay proper treatment or result in misdiagnosis. Difficulty pinning down the actual problem in the elderly can occur with any illness, not just serious ones such as heart attack or appendicitis. One theory called "weakest link" claims that any illness can manifest itself as failure of that person's weakest organ system. For instance, some elderly people become confused or delirious when they develop a lung infection yet show few typical signs of pneumonia. Others might become incontinent of urine as a first sign of some illness remote from the bladder.

With all the risks for elderly patients one would imagine that doctors would do everything possible to avoid hospitalizing these patients, particularly frail nursing home patients. Alarmingly, nearly half of acute hospitalizations of nursing home residents may be inappropriate, according to a recent study published in the *Journal of the American Geriatric Society*.[30] In fact, this study found a close association between inappropriate transfer to an emergency room (or hospitalization) and poor quality of care. When a frail and chronically ill patient is trans-ferred to an emergency room, the treating ER doctor is usually unfa-miliar with that patient. That doctor might mistakenly believe the patient is acutely ill when in reality much of the illness is baseline or an ongoing condition. Rather than treating a minor problem like a urinary tract infection and sending the patient back to the nursing home, that person ends up hospitalized until the primary care doctor sorts things out.

In truth, chronic illnesses like congestive heart failure usually occur gradually. Many nursing home patients could avoid hospitalization or an emergency room visit with closer supervision at the nursing home, according to a health policy report on emergency department use by nursing home residents.[31]

Unfamiliar Patients at Risk

Have you neglected to see your physician for more than a year or two? Or have you not yet met your primary care doctor, a common scenario with managed care insurance plans? If you have not made an effort to establish a relationship with your doctor, he or she will not feel any obligation to you as an absentee patient. An ongoing relationship between physician and patient including regular visits creates a healer-patient bond. Without that bond, you are more likely to be subjected to a "lazy admission."

You will also become an "unfamiliar" patient if you fall ill while on vacation or while traveling away from home. If you should need admis-sion into the hospital, the on-call doctor covering the emergency department will not know you. That doctor may well employ the "lazy admission" if you require a hospital stay. More than likely, your plan of care will not be double-checked and you will not get that extra hand-holding and reassurance.

Uninsured or "Service Patients" at Risk

Patients who are on public assistance or those with no insurance are con-sidered to be "service patients" by healthcare professionals. The admit-ting physician rarely makes a special trip into the hospital to fulfill the three primary patient needs for these individuals. The reasoning: "My pay will be a pittance, if anything at all, so why not let the emergency doctor or intern do the work since they are already at the hospital." The more experienced doctor will not be there to provide words of comfort and careful thought to the diagnosis and treatment plan.

WHEN ONE DOCTOR "COVERS" ANOTHER DOCTOR

On any given night, Doctor A "covers" the patients of Doctor B so Doctor B can have uninterrupted personal time. Another night or weekend, Doctor B will cover for Doctor A. The covering physician might be a partner, colleague or friend of the off-duty physician. If there is a problem with the off-duty doctor's patient, the covering physician must care for that patient. If the covering physician does not know you, chances are good he or she will not want to commence a relationship with you the night you become ill. The lazy admission might well be used if you require (or seem to require) hospitalization. That means either the emergency room doctor will write quick orders to admit you or an inexperienced intern will write the orders. The unfamiliar (covering) doctor might spend little or no time on your behalf.

Hospitals are clearly not hotels and each night you stay brings added risk. We are all at risk for the "lazy admission." Now you can learn how to avoid it.

AVOIDING THE "LAZY ADMISSION"

You've heard it before: The hospital is the worst place to be if you are sick. Believe it, it's true! Before you check into the heart-disease hotel, ask your doctor if admission into the hospital is absolutely essential or just a precaution. Remember, the final decision to move from the emergency room to a hospital room rests in the patient's hands.

GUIDELINES FOR AGREEING
TO BE ADMITTED INTO THE HOSPITAL

1. Ask your doctor how strongly he or she feels about you staying in the hospital. If your doctor firmly and confidently says leaving would risk life or limb, then stay! If your doctor sounds unsure, consider leaving. For example, if you have a mild kidney infection and your doctor says (in so many words), "Well, your white blood cell count is 16.5 thousand and the protocol is to admit a patient if it's higher than 16 thousand...." Your answer: "See ya. I'm outta here! I'll send you a postcard when I finish the antibiotics." The key question is "What can be done for me in the hospital that could not be done if I went home?"

2. Be more skeptical about being admitted into the hospital by a covering doctor, particularly one who did not actually examine you in the emergency department. Also, if an intern (young training doctor) makes the admitting decision (you *will* ask who is treating you

at a teaching hospital), be sure an attending physician speaks to you to give you a more experienced explanation and opinion.

3. Get opinions from the senior emergency room doctor and your family doctor on the need for you to be hospitalized. If both doctors agree that you need to stay in the hospital, it is probably true.
4. If you have any other risk factors or health problems that make the immediate problem potentially more dangerous, leaving may invite unnecessary risk.

Ask all doctors and consulting specialists what the realistic risks are of being cared for as an outpatient, including careful follow up. If the cardiologist, for instance, is truly concerned that your vague chest pains could be a heart problem, he might tell you sudden heart attack or death are real concerns. Then stay. If doctors tell you there is a remote risk something bad might happen, they should also tell you *staying* in the hospital poses a higher than remote risk of complications. If hospital admission is simply a precaution (translation: "let's avoid malpractice risk"), then politely decline the invitation to be admitted.

Additional Tips for Successful Hospital Admissions:

- Remember the Rule of Three: When you are being admitted into the hospital, you need *reassurance*, *explanation* and a solid, safe *game plan* for proper diagnosis, relief of discomfort and cure.
- Never say, "Whatever you say, doc." It should be reflexive for you or your advocate to ask if hospital admission or testing can be avoided.
- Maintain a close and honest relationship with your family doctor. Visit your doctor regularly for checkups even when feeling well. This is a good way to avoid "physician-phobia," a phrase I use to describe the irrational fear that your doctor will *make* you sick by simply diagnosing an illness you already have. If you visit your doctor's office in good health, you will usually return home robust as well. It is vital to practice *preventive* medical care to detect illness early—before it becomes serious. When you fall ill, your family doctor becomes your best friend and ally. That bond between physician and patient is what someday will get your doctor out of bed at three A.M. to properly care for you in the emergency room.

DANGER #12
GURNEY GRIDLOCK

Picture people on stretchers lining busy hallways, two or three stuffed behind a curtain like sardines packed in a can. Envision patients in dark corridor corners with little supervision. Visualize some people right in the center of the emergency department on display like a sofa in a department store. These images are not horror scenes in a sensationalized doctor drama. They might be happening at your local emergency department.

"Gurney gridlock" is a serious problem in our overcrowded emergency rooms. Urban hospitals might have as many as thirty patients being held in the emergency department, because no beds are available in the hospital, particularly the coveted intensive care and heart monitoring beds. These patients remain on hard stretchers in the emergency department sometimes for days, subjected to constant noise and hubbub. This is hardly the way to control blood pressure or recuperate from a heart attack.

AMBULANCE DIVERSION

Overcrowding in our health care centers leads to a chain reaction of dangerous events. Hospital beds and intensive care units fill up. With no place to go, new patients in the emergency department who require observation or hospital admission are stuck in the emergency department. When the ER holds many patients in an observation area or in hallways, nursing and doctor shortages are felt more acutely. The emergency department becomes dangerously overwhelmed so the next step is for the ER to go on "ambulance diversion." That means ambulances cannot transport any more patients—even the most severely ill—to that hospital. Sick patients cannot go to the hospital where their doctors send them. Instead, they must ride around in an ambulance until some hospital gives them the okay and once a patient does arrive after a delay that emergency room is usually in a state of sheer chaos. This is hardly the place someone wants to be for quality care. During peak busy seasons such as winter flu epidemics, it is not unusual for several big city hospitals in a community to be on "ambulance diversion" simultaneously!

What is so bad about being stretcher-bound in a hallway in a busy emergency room for many hours to a few days? As long as you're getting proper care, you'll live through it, you think. Not that simple. Along with overcrowding, inevitably comes chaos and neglect. Inadequate staffing with properly trained nurses to closely monitor seriously ill patients adds to the dangers. Physicians might check on their patients for only minutes in a day, if at all. The consequences can be catastrophic. The woman with heart failure might re-accumulate water in her lungs; the stroke patient's blood pressure might soar; the senile man might fall from a stretcher when a side rail is accidently left down. It is not rare for patients to be found dead on hallway stretchers in chaotic emergency rooms! Your goal as a patient is to avoid becoming part of such hallway havoc and a recipient of the slapdash care that follows.

STEERING CLEAR OF GURNEY GRIDLOCK

You need to be admitted into the hospital and you are stuck in the emergency room. No beds are available in the hospital. Nurses whiz by like cars on a freeway. Doctors' voices seem to echo across the ER in loud monotones. Carts and machinery squeak and scrape past you at regular intervals. Your care might be compromised when you are caught in the chaotic web of a busy emergency department. Emergency room workers become distracted. There are not enough doctors and nurses to carefully monitor all patients. Miscommunications occur and orders and treatments are delayed or forgotten.

Drs. Derlet and Richards, in their article about emergency department overcrowding published in the *Annals of Emergency Medicine*, propose several ideal solutions to the dangerous overcrowding problem:

1. Better access to clinics for both insured and uninsured patients.
2. Expanding inpatient hospital bed capabilities, particularly intensive care and heart monitoring beds.
3. Developing specialized ER observation units.
4. Expanding emergency doctor, nursing, and ancillary staff.
5. Building larger emergency departments with more bed space.
6. Improving the support of radiology, laboratory, and consultant services.

These solutions are unlikely to be implemented any time soon, because at this time, for hospital administrators, cost containment takes precedence over enhancing patient care. Without these solutions, Drs. Derlet and Richards predict that overcrowding will grow worse. "The general public may no longer be able to rely on emergency departments for quality and timely emergency care, placing the safety of people in this country at risk," they write.[32]

What can you do to minimize your chances of getting stuck sleeping in the emergency room for one or more nights? There are several options that might be available to you:

- Politely pressure your family doctor to get you a bed. Do not immediately adopt an attitude of resignation. Being sick is hard enough so you do not need your health jeopardized as well. Every hospital can at times have "invisible" beds available. These beds might be concealed by floor staff to avoid another admission or reserved for another doctor's patient who is arriving later as an elective admission. If your doctor presses the issue at the admitting office, a bed might suddenly appear. Your doctor, however, might not have enough clout to secure an invisible bed.

- Use as your family doctor a physician who has clout in the hospital. The chairman or associate director of a department or the physician in charge of the intensive care unit is more likely to get a scarce bed for you by throwing some weight around. For instance, patients are often kept in scarce monitored beds, but do not require that high-level care. Their physician put them there "just in case." The doctor in charge of these beds can have that "just-in-case" patient moved out to make room for you, his or her patient.

- If the first two options are not possible, ask your doctor to transfer you to another facility that has beds available. Many physicians have admitting privileges at more than one hospital. If your doctor does not work at other hospitals, he or she can refer you to a colleague at that other hospital.

- Your final option is to accept your stay in the emergency room. You might get a bed soon if three patients are being held in gurney gridlock, but if ten or twenty patients are awaiting beds then you have a problem of long duration.

Once sentenced to a lengthy stay in the emergency department, prepare yourself in advance. If you might need the urinal or bedpan soon, for instance, ask for it before you actually have to use it. The most important times to plan ahead are during shift changes for doctors and nurses. Most commonly, changeover occurs at 7:00 or 8:00 o'clock, day or night. Other common times for staff changeover could be 3:00 or 4:00 in the afternoon and 11:00 or 12:00 at night. It is virtually impossible to get anything for fifteen to thirty minutes during shift changes. Anticipate these times when you feel you might need assistance soon. If your pain or nausea is returning, ask for the next dose of medication thirty minutes in advance of the shift change. This is emergency room survival. Most importantly, if you are in trouble—chest pain has returned or breathing is worse—call out for help. Yell! Do not be shy! It can be hard to flag down a nurse or doctor in the busy emergency department. Stay alert during the day, but ask for a potent sleeping pill to get needed rest at night.

DANGER #13
ATTITUDES THAT DESTROY
DOCTOR-PATIENT RELATIONSHIPS

Can a patient trust the emergency doctor's concern and desire to help when the first words from the doctor's mouth are, "What's so urgent that you need to be here at 3:00 A.M.?" Surely a patient loses faith in the compassion of medical workers when the nurse says to someone with a severe headache, "Why are you moaning like there's a stick of dynamite in your head?" A patient loses trust in her healers after overhearing nurses and doctors joke, "She's had the symptoms for a week, couldn't she wait one day more until I'm off?" or "She's probably crying for attention," or "Another stupid mother, not first giving her baby fever-reducing medication." Will patients follow instructions and comply with medication if they mistrust their caretakers? A sensitive patient might tune out after hearing a derisive remark, thereby misunderstanding important instructions.

Patients might encounter sarcastic remarks from desk clerk to doctor during an emergency room visit. In addition to sarcasm, there are many other disdainful attitudes to which patients might fall victim. The following negative attitudes are commonly encountered in emergency rooms. They breed hostility and blow gaping holes through the healer-patient relationship. The result is a hemorrhaging of trust from vulnerable patients.

THE EUREKA PHENOMENON

Patients who seek care at an emergency room for minor or chronic problems are subjected to hostility and sarcasm, particularly during busy times. They will often encounter a riptide of hurried care, leading them out the exit door from the moment they enter the ER. Why *do* patients come to emergency rooms with chronic or minor problems? There are three common reasons: no family physician, a physician who is away or a primary care doctor who is not available on short notice. Surely it is reasonable to go to an emergency room if chronic symptoms suddenly get much worse. In many cases, however, there are no easy explanations as to why someone seeks emergency care for chronic or minor medical problems.

I call this enigma the "Eureka Phenomenon," and it describes that moment of decision when a person decides to seek help from emergency caregivers. That moment may come after days of pain, weeks of discomfort or months of recurrent symptoms, but it is that one moment of enlightenment that defines this phenomenon. Such revelations often seem to come at two o'clock in the morning. Consider the following examples of this odd and perplexing phenomenon:

A woman calls the emergency room at 11:00 P.M. and asks if she should rush her son in. The reason: He has had an ingrown toenail for one week. He is twenty years old. In another Eureka moment of realization, a young man tells the emergency doctor at 1:00 A.M. that his lower back has been aching for two months. In a third instance of this phenomenon, a man describes an aching sensation in his legs that gets aggravated each time he works a long day at the factory. He has had these pains for five years and wonders if he might be eligible for disability. He has never tried a household pain reliever. What can explain her epiphany when a woman arrives at the ER and complains that she has a cockroach in her ear and wants it removed? She casually tells the doctor it has been there for a long time!

During a quiet night, the "Eureka patient" interrupts the doctor or nurse from much needed sleep and the clerk and nursing assistants from intriguing conversations and catching up on their paperwork. During busy times, "Eureka patients" turn an already hectic atmosphere into sheer chaos and distract attention away from seriously ill patients. "Eureka patients" with chronic problems are always an unwelcome burden to emergency staff. Healthcare professionals, like anybody else, instinctively react with sarcasm or hostility toward burdens perceived as unnecessary and unwanted.

The "Eureka Phenomenon" is not simply a benign curiosity or inconvenience. Patients may be at great risk from this type of treatment-seeking behavioral pattern. First, the hostility and scorn the "Eureka patient" elicits might shatter the physician or nurse-patient relationship. Patients, feeling insulted and criticized, are less likely to comply with follow-up care and instructions. Second, physicians and nurses are more likely to miss serious illnesses in their early stages by not taking seriously even trivial or longstanding complaints. For example, one week of abdominal pain in a healthy looking elderly man could have been dismissed as nothing of importance: it turned out to be a ruptured appendix. Under emergency room crunch conditions, the seriousness of indigestion-type pains for a few days might be minimized without considering a heart attack or gallbladder attack. One primary function of emergency care, after all, is to "rule out" or exclude the presence of serious or life-threatening illness.

Lastly, adding insult to injury, the "Eureka patient" will get charged full price for the emergency room visit even after a cursory evaluation. Imagine the frustration: A three-hour wait for a three minute evaluation and that patient will be sent back to his or her family doctor—the place to which the patient should have gone first.

"Eureka patients'" complaints are often dismissed as psychiatric problems or as being trivial without careful evaluation by the ER staff. On the other end of the spectrum, some of these patients might get useless X rays or tests for a truly minor problem just because they sought care at an emergency room.

ASSORTED DETRIMENTAL ATTITUDES

The "He deserves what he gets" reaction can be cruel. This mind-set is directed at those patients who have self-inflicted disease or injury from drug abuse or violence. A man who breaks his hand punching the wall while aiming for his wife's face might be kept waiting an extra hour or two without pain medicine.

There is also the "She or he's a complainer" outlook toward patients, usually elderly, who have multiple complaints and frequent flier mileage to the emergency room. The term "GOMER" has been used for years to describe old, sickly patients with many medical problems. The acronym stands for "Get Out of My Emergency Room." These patients might have a serious illness the one time emergency workers do not take them seriously. What's more, many of these patients sense they are being mocked. Not only is their dignity lost, so is their faith in the medical profession. No wonder they comply poorly with their treatment.

The "He or she's just a drug seeker" condemnation might deprive someone of pain medication who is truly suffering, when strong pain medicine is withheld. No test exists which can measure degree of pain.

The "histrionics" or "hysteria" attitude (sometimes referred to as "ay-ay-ay" or "oy-oy-oy") implies that anyone who violently gesticulates or yells must not be truly sick or in pain and is only overreacting. This is cruel treatment for someone with a migraine headache or who is passing a kidney stone, for instance. Studies have found that Hispanic and African-American ER patients were less likely than non-minority patients to get medication to treat pain. Also, younger patients were more likely to receive pain medication than elderly patients. Such results indicate that pain treatment, possibly all treatments, may be subjective and influenced by more than the patient's symptoms and medical history.

If a doctor quickly labels a patient as "hysterical," the consequences can be devastating. Consider a frightening case that was published in an emergency medicine journal section called "Avoidable Errors."[33] A nineteen year-old woman was brought to a *third* emergency room for a complaint of "I can barely move anything." The first two emergency rooms sent her home with the recommendation to seek psychiatric help for hysteria. The emergency room doctor at the third ER did a cursory examination after observing the young woman's detached behavior, a demeanor that is characteristic of hysteria. The doctor asked her to lift her legs and thought her inability to do so was exaggerated. She asked in a calm, unconcerned tone, "Doctor, do you think I will ever walk again?" Like the other two, this doctor concluded she was hysterical based on an attitude he had about her behavior. Another doctor in the emergency room saw her and suspected she might be truly ill while the first doctor was arranging for her rapid discharge. That night, she stopped breathing and needed to be on a breathing machine until she recovered several months later. She suffered from a life-threatening complication of a viral infection called Guillain-Barre. Thankfully, that astute doctor, the fourth to see her, did keep her in the hospital that day. Negative attitudes can surely do more damage than simply hurting a patient's feelings.

AVOIDING ANTAGONISTIC ATTITUDES

Follow these rules and your trip to the emergency room can be more rewarding and pleasant. You might even get better care.

1. *Hostility Alienates.* Be polite and patient, but keep on top of things. When was the last time your boss gleefully gave you a raise after you called him a cheap bum? Don't expect smiles from the emergency room staff after similar behavior. Your care can suffer if doctors and nurses avoid you because of rude behavior from yourself or your family. ER workers are, after all, human and will harbor personal resentments or hostilities toward a rude or unreasonably demanding person.

2. *Don't Be a "Eureka Patient."* If at all possible, avoid emergency room visits for less serious problems that you have had longer than two or three days. Call your family doctor and urge him or her to fit you into office hours. Walk-in facilities such as urgent care centers can be a good alternative. Remember, "Eureka patients" receive hurried, shoddy care at premium prices. A three-minute, in-and-out examination for abdominal

pain or severe back pain present for several days is no guarantee that all is okay!

3. *Stupidity Infuriates.* Caring for the ill is a hard job. Do not make it harder on medical personnel. Try common sense remedies and first aid before rushing to an emergency room. Buy a reputable first aid reference book. Call your family physician for advice. Some examples: For fever, take the temperature first then use acetaminophen or ibuprofen in proper doses; for pain, try ibuprofen or acetaminophen as well; for bleeding, elevate the area and put direct pressure on the wound to stop bleeding (it might take twenty to thirty minutes); for diarrhea in a healthy adult or older child, drink liquids, avoid milk products and try constipating measures such as rice, bananas or an over-the-counter diarrhea remedy. If symptoms persist, first call your doctor for additional suggestions before heading to the ER.

4. *Bring a Voice of Reason.* You are in pain or scared or vomiting. It is hard to remain cool and calm. You simply do not take well to discomfort. You become grumpy. Does that mean you should be shunned or mocked or ignored in the emergency room? No, but it might happen. So bring along a friend or relative who can calmly explain to emergency staff what you feel, what you need and that you do not normally behave that way.

5. *Pick Your Spots.* Be selective. Do not demand everything. If you complain vociferously about each and every problem, no one will take you seriously. Emergency staff will avoid and resent you. Demand only important things such as promptly being given medication for pain.

6. *Plan Ahead.* While it is reasonable to expect prompt solutions to important problems, do not assume someone will be instantly available to do so. This is particularly true if a critically ill patient arrives and ties up many ER workers. It is prudent to plan requests in advance. Ask for pain medication *before* the previous dose has fully worn off. Be certain you have a bedpan available if you cannot walk to a bathroom. Ask for a sleeping pill before the change of shift and hold on to it if you want to stay awake a short while longer.

DANGER #14
BEING RIPPED-OFF AT THE ER REGISTER

Do you clip coupons? Watch the supermarket cashier like a hawk? Go to garage sales? Shop around? Like a preacher adheres to the word of the Bible, many consumers abide by these "rules" and others like them to help make ends meet. Despite consumer savvy, many people squander large amounts of money on medical care. For instance, many people are penny wise and dollar foolish. They might delay needed medical care if they must pay for it and then wind up with a far more serious and costly problem because of the delay. The older adult with a bad cough and fever should not avoid spending two hundred dollars for an office evaluation only to wind up hospitalized with a serious lung infection because of the delay.

There are other examples of lack of consumer savvy with regard to healthcare. Ask a former patient what tests were done during an emergency room visit and they might stare at you blankly. Do you call several pharmacies or medical supply stores to get the lowest price for medication or supplies? A Web search might save you money for medical supplies or medication if you buy these from a reputable online company.

Like any store or supermarket bill, errors are common on emergency department or hospital bills. In fact, over ninety percent of hospital bills reviewed by Congress's General Accounting Office had errors! There is no cash register screen to watch as medical expenses pile up during your ER visit. Several varieties of money squandering are common in the emergency room or hospital setting:

- Unnecessary ER Visits
- Clerical Errors
- Repeated, Refused or Cancelled Tests
- High Markups and Overcharges
- Too Many Cooks in the ER Kitchen
- Killing an Ant with a Sledgehammer

Unnecessary Emergency Room Visits

Your first step in spending money wisely is to ask yourself and then your family doctor, "Is an emergency room visit truly necessary?" The amount you are charged for care in an emergency room can be double what it actually costs in a non-emergency setting, according to researchers at the University of Michigan. The one hundred percent markup compensates the hospital for its losses from treating patients who cannot or will not pay. What can you do in a pinch when the injury or illness is not limb or life threatening? Other options for care include simple home remedies under your doctor's guidance, an office visit to your family doctor within twelve to twenty-four hours or an immediate visit to an urgent care facility. Any of these choices are likely to be less expensive than an emergency room visit (average ER fee just to register to be evaluated is about $250 to $500). Will a visit to an urgent care facility be appropriate for your problem? Does the urgent care facility accept your insurance or will you have to pay out of pocket? These are issues you must sort out in advance so you do not have to squander money during an illness. In addition, a phone call to your family doctor might help to clarify borderline problems and thus steer you to the proper health care facility.

Clerical Errors

Typos are harmless on paper except when they appear on your emergency room or hospital bill. Clerical errors can cost you hundreds of dollars. Double billing for a medication, supply or test is a common mistake. Someone else's test or treatment might be written on your chart and you'll be charged for it. Diagnosis codes are numerical representations of the diseases with which patients are diagnosed. If someone enters the wrong number, a minor ailment might be transformed into a serious and expensive one. Similarly, when hospitals code for tests or procedures using numbers, one typo could turn a simple test that was actually performed into an expensive test that is entered on the bill.

Another common error is to enter the wrong number of days you were in the ER or hospital. Some hospitals will even bill you for a full day if you are admitted into the hospital at ten or eleven P.M. Remain alert, too, for billing entries that charge you for a service not provided. For example, did you actually get the five hours of recovery room observation listed on the bill? Did you receive that heart monitoring or oxygen therapy? The only way to find these errors is to maintain a careful record while you are in the ER or hospital and to compare your records to an itemized, plain English bill of charges.

Repeated, Refused or Cancelled Tests

Tests often go awry. They get screwed up. Blood samples might get "hemolyzed" which means blood cells were damaged during collection or handling of the sample. Blood tests also mysteriously disappear (perhaps the messenger dropped it?). Blood can clot in the test tube. Laboratory tests must be repeated when the computerized machine gives an inaccurate readout or perhaps an unexpectedly abnormal result. Lastly, a doctor's afterthought may mean more blood needs to be drawn to run additional tests.

Electrocardiograms give zigzag readouts of the electrical workings of the heart. Sometimes the machine zags before it zigs and another electrocardiogram must be done. X rays are frequently repeated for technical problems as well. If the technologist "misfires" the X ray, it might be undercooked (too light) or overdone (too dark) making it difficult to interpret accurately. Extra views might be added to an X-ray study that has a fixed price. Find out if you are being charged for special X-ray views for the doctor's convenience (comparison films of a child's normal ankle, for instance).

Sometimes tests are ordered and then cancelled if a patient refuses a test after a discussion with the physician or if the physician decides that test is not needed. A charge for that test may, nevertheless, show up on your bill, even though it was cancelled. There are many ways for a bill to end up with mistaken charges, particularly in a hectic emergency department, therefore you or your advocate must be vigilant about keeping track of your ER treatment.

High Markups and Overcharges

Hospitals often charge ridiculously high markups on supplies and equipment. Charging $20.00 for a gauze dressing or toothbrush is not unusual. Charging $15.00 for only two ibuprofen tablets seems a little inappropriate. Some hospitals defend these charges as "the cost of doing business." Such markups, they claim, simply compensate for their losses from nonpaying patients.

At times, a hospital might bill separately for several supplies that were in one prepackaged kit. The individual charges can be considerably higher. Patients can usually negotiate to have some of these charges removed or corrected.

Too Many Cooks in the ER Kitchen

Many family physicians will call in a specialist for virtually everything. An expert opinion is great, but it can cost you big bucks. Be a skeptic and look at it as too many cooks in the medical care kitchen before you agree to call in a specialist. Is it truly needed? Ask both your family and emergency room doctors what their reasoning is. You might consider changing your family doctor if he cannot handle *basic* problems without calling upon a specialist. On the other hand, be wary of a doctor who believes he alone can handle everything.

Additional hidden costs exist for specialist assistance, about which you should be aware. Not only will you pay for an electrocardiogram, but also for an expert reading of that test by a cardiologist who reads every electrocardiogram that gets done in the emergency room. The same holds true for X-ray studies. Expect a separate bill from a radiologist who officially interpreted that test.

Killing an Ant With a Sledgehammer

Kill an ant with a sledgehammer and you'll find mass destruction beneath the bug. Try swatting a fly with a baseball bat and the wall beneath will crumble in the process. There are consequences to each doctor's approach to treating an illness. Avoid big risks that offer small gains. Even if no harm befalls you, treatment overkill can be costly. Taking a potent antibiotic for minor illness serves as a useful example. For instance, why spend one hundred dollars for an antibiotic when ten dollars of penicillin will be effective for "strep throat." Avoid designer anti-inflammatory pain medicines when generic aspirin or ibuprofen will do as well. To take it one step further, that potent antibiotic might cause a yeast infection or bad diarrhea that can lead to even more ailments and treatments. That new designer anti-inflammatory medication might be the one that gives you a stomach ulcer. Try to stick with old reliable treatments that have been shown to be safe, well tolerated and effective. Keep things simple.

HOW TO BE A SMART MEDICAL AID SHOPPER

These emergency care shopping tips will help you to save money and become a wise healthcare consumer:

1. Choose your emergency room visits carefully. It is less expensive to go to an urgent care center or physician's office for ailments which are less serious or a few days old.

2. Always jot down all tests and treatments performed and those that are cancelled. If you are too ill, then have your friend or relative keep a log. The bill might come weeks later, at which time your recall will be vague. It is good practice for a patient to know exactly what tests were done and those results, as well as any treatments given (see ER Visit Log in Appendix D).

3. Bluntly ask your private or emergency doctor if that specialist

is really needed. Remember, too, that with specialist consultations often come additional tests and procedures.

4. Stock your medicine chest well so you can avoid wasteful emergency visits to relieve sudden pain, itch, diarrhea, vomiting or other common symptoms. Those who have a history of a wrenched back or kidney stone, for instance, should have an ample supply of effective pain medication from their family doctor should an attack strike at odd hours. If you get migraine headaches, be sure to have a stock of an effective medication. Order medications in bulk if you must use them for three months or more.

5. Ask how much the prescription that the emergency room doctor convinces you will be beneficial will cost. Request the least expensive and safest choice. Some doctors use newfangled versions of medications which might be expensive and the toxicity of which might not yet be known. Some doctors are affected by drug company advertising and you might be the guinea pig on whom they are trying these new medications. There are, however, some difficult or resistant infections that will need a more potent antibiotic. If you *do* need the pharmaceutical sledgehammer approach, call several pharmacies for pricing. You might be amazed by the wide price variation.

6. Request a fully itemized bill, in plain English and not code numbers, from the hospital or emergency department. The "miscellaneous" category should be itemized as well. If necessary, your doctor can help to clarify which tests, treatments or supplies were indeed used.

7. After reviewing the bill, if you have any questions contact the emergency room or hospital Billing or Patient Accounts Department. If they will not help to resolve your concerns, you can try the hospital's Patient Advocate (or Representative).

8. Consider using a claims assistance company. These companies will negotiate with emergency rooms, doctors or hospitals to get you a better deal or to simply remove any mistaken charges. Call the Alliance of Claims Assistance Professionals (ACAP) for information or a recommendation at 1-877-275-8765. Also, try Medical Billing Advocates of America at 540-387-5870.

9. Notify your insurance company within two days after an emergency room visit if your insurance company requires it. Many insurance companies have relaxed their strict regulation of

emergency room visits but be alert to the rules of your policy. The reason: At least thirty-three states have enacted "Prudent Lay Person" laws that require an insurance company to pay for any emergency room visit for problems that an average person would have thought could be an emergency. For instance, if your chest pain turns out to be just indigestion from the chili you devoured last night, your insurance company must still pay for heart testing and any other evaluation. Learn now if your state has a "Prudent Lay Person" law.

USEFUL WEB SITES

http://www.claims.org

(The Alliance of Claims Assistance Professionals provides information to members and referrals to healthcare consumers in need of claims assistance.)

http://www.healthallies.com

(Health Allies is an online service that helps individuals find affordable healthcare services whether they are insured and uninsured.)

http://www.billadvocates.com

(Medical Billing Advocates of America work with healthcare consumers to reduce the cost of expensive medical bills by deciphering charges, detecting errors and maximizing insurance reimbursements.)

PART

3

PROPER USE
OF THE EMERGENCY ROOM

SHOULD YOU GO TO THE ER?

By now you might be thinking you do not want to set foot in an emergency room as long as you live. That would be unwise and unrealistic. Knowing the flaws in our emergency care system, you are now better prepared to sidestep emergency room dangers and use the emergency room safely. After all, emergency care *does* save many lives.

When you fall ill many questions come to mind. Do I need to see a doctor? Should I try an over-the-counter remedy? Which one? How do I know if my illness is serious?

Basic guidelines to follow should sudden medical illness strike:

1. *Are the symptoms unbearable?* If so, seek help immediately. If symptoms are tolerable and you can perform your normal activities then ask yourself...

2. *How long have symptoms lasted?* If you've had them on and off for one or more days, you are probably safer than if severe symptoms came on suddenly and persistently at the outset. Then ask yourself...

3. *Have I ever had the same symptoms before?* Do I have any serious health problems that might be related? If symptoms are familiar, you might know the remedy from past experience. Many people will self-treat their recurrent indigestion with antacids, for example. Women are often familiar with the symptoms of urinary tract infections. If you are older than fifty or suffer from serious chronic illness such as high blood pressure, diabetes or heart problems you should be more cautious about feeling ill. Then ask...

125

4. *Is this by far the worst* headache, difficulty breathing, abdominal pain or other symptom I've ever experienced? If so, seek professional advice or immediate help. If symptoms do not stop you from continuing your daily routine, try simple measures.

5. *Have I tried simple remedies* such as antacids or a pain reliever? If two acetaminophen (Tylenol) or ibuprofen (anti-inflammatory household pain remedy) relieve your headache it is less likely to be serious. If an antacid definitely relieves your abdominal discomfort or heartburn, there is less cause for concern.

If symptoms are unbearable, go to an emergency room without delay. For worst-ever symptoms that are bearable, those that persist for several hours (or days) or those unrelieved by simple remedies, it is time to call your family doctor (if you have one, otherwise seek immediate medical care). People who have chronic medical illnesses such as diabetes and those over age fifty should err on the side of caution about an unfamiliar or unexplainable ill feeling. Call your doctor for advice.

When your doctor (or the covering associate) returns your call, describe your symptoms, relevant past medical history, medications you take and remedies you tried that day. The doctor will then give you one of three suggestions:

1. "Don't worry. Continue simple remedies."
2. "Come into the office today or tomorrow for an examination."
3. "Get medical care now at an emergency room or urgent care office."

If your doctor does not answer your call within thirty minutes or if you are feeling worse, seek medical care at an urgent care center or emergency room.

THE TEN COMMANDMENTS
OF THE EMERGENCY ROOM

If you are headed to the emergency room heed and obey these Ten Commandments or suffer the consequences!

I. *Thou shalt plan in advance your emergency rooms of choice.* Do not try to decide during a crisis. Learn which hospitals are best for trauma, pediatric and heart care. Do proper research. Know each hospital's limitations and strong points. Ask your doctor at which hospital he or she has admitting privileges or use a doctor who holds admitting privileges at a university hospital. Map out the shortest drive to those hospitals.

II. *Never delay seeking help* for unfamiliar or severe chest pain, shortness of breath, abdominal pain, limb numbness or weakness and worst-ever headache. Have someone notify your doctor while you wait for an ambulance. Do not drive yourself to a hospital if suffering such symptoms.

III. *Know thy emergency physician.* Ask if he or she completed training and in what field. Is the doctor a full-time emergency room physician? A moonlighter? Don't be shy. Ask. Your well-being may depend on it!

IV. *Know thy medicines and their dosages.* Carry an updated list in your wallet or bring the bottles with you to the emergency room. Over-the-counter remedies like aspirin or antacids are also medications. Herbal remedies and vitamins should also be mentioned.

V. *Thou shalt carry in thy wallet a laminated, miniaturized copy of your electrocardiogram.* This is key if you have a heart condition or are over fifty years of age. The diagnosis of a heart attack does not always jump off the electrocardiogram. The best way to diagnose heart trouble is to compare a new electrocardiogram with a previous one to detect changes.

VI. *Never consent to any test, treatment, or procedure* unless the doctor clearly explains its purpose and the associated risks versus benefits. Politely ask if safer alternatives exist and if the test is truly needed. It is your right as patient to refuse a test.

VII. *Thou shalt not worship X rays, blood tests, medications or doctors.* Avoid high-tech, pill-popping or white-coat idolatry; kneel only to compassion and common sense.

VIII. *Thou shalt stick with one hospital (and doctor) when possible.* Access to old records can help to avoid needless repetition of tests and provide important information for physicians and nurses. The exception: For serious pediatric and heart illness or severe injury go to the best-equipped hospital as well as the most skilled and experienced doctor.

IX. *Thou shalt not make threats or demands toward emergency staff.* Never mention the phrase "law suit." Politely ask and inquire. Do not demand and challenge or thou shall be spurned and ostracized.

X. *Avoid emergency room visits for problems that have been present three days or longer.* These non-emergencies should be handled in a doctor's office or urgent care center. Your doctor can send you to the hospital should you require hospitalization. An exception to the three-day rule: if symptoms dramatically worsen on the third day, then seeking emergency room care is appropriate.

RED FLAGS:
POSSIBLE SYMPTOMS AND
AND SIGNS OF SERIOUS PROBLEMS

Each person experiences illness in a unique way. Every person has a different pain threshold. What's more, not every heart or appendix attack happens in a textbook fashion. Some people might work through the pain and leave it untreated; others will rush to seek help at the first twinge of discomfort. The elderly and children often do not have typical symptoms for many illnesses, which can muddy the diagnostic waters. The following section discusses telltale signs that suggest a more serious problem is brewing.

CHEST PAIN

Five people describe having chest pains. One is cured by the surgical procedure called balloon angioplasty, the second is cured with antacids, the third with a sedative, the fourth with ibuprofen and the last with antibiotics. Why are there five totally different cures for similar chest pains? Chest pain is one of medicine's great riddles. Many different body organs can send or refer pain to the chest area including the heart, stomach, food tube, ribs, muscles, lungs and even the brain! Because physicians cannot easily discern the true cause for chest pain, patients should maintain healthy skepticism if a doctor gives a snap diagnosis. Inquire how the doctor arrived at that conclusion. Did the doctor perform an electrocardiogram (EKG) in an effort to rule out a heart problem? Your risk factors for heart disease and the nature of symptoms can help determine a high or low probability that your chest pains are heart-related—one of the most serious causes for chest pain.

Major Risk Factors For Heart Disease:
- Older age
- Having parents or siblings with heart attacks or heart disease before age sixty
- Smoking cigarettes
- Having diabetes

- Having high blood pressure
- Prior angina or heart attack
- Having high blood levels of bad cholesterol or triglycerides

Additional Risk Factors For Heart Problems:
- Illegal drug use such as cocaine or amphetamines
- Obesity
- Sedentary life style
- Stress

Do you imagine a heart attack (myocardial infarction) sufferer to be an overweight, stressed out, middle-aged man who suddenly develops crushing chest pain then collapses to the ground? You are not alone. Portrayal of heart attacks in the media and Hollywood can be misleading since most heart attacks are not so dramatic. Heart attacks frequently cause slowly progressive and vague symptoms. In fact, as many as one-third of heart attacks do not even cause any chest pain!

Another misconception is that women are at lower risk than men for heart disease. While it is true that women generally have heart attacks at older ages than men, heart disease ranks as the leading cause of death in both men and women.

Why is all this so important? Many people have misconceptions about their risk for heart attack and may lack knowledge of the less typical symptoms commonly experienced by sufferers. These people are at great risk of ignoring warning signs and delaying seeking care for a heart attack, care that is highly time-dependent and can save lives with early treatment. Recall that "time is muscle."

Emergency room factors that contribute to treatment delays are difficult enough to deal with (see Danger #1), but when patients themselves delay seeking treatment a bad outcome is even more tragic. Averting death, disability, and suffering can be in every person's hands. Effective clot-dissolving treatment is available to stop a heart attack in its tracks if given within one to three hours after symptoms begin. After three to six hours the benefits no longer justify the dangers inherent in the treatment.

The first step is for people to become familiar with *all* heart attack symptoms. Doctors, too, must be more alert to subtle signs of heart disease. Less typical symptoms are more likely to mislead doctors, particularly those who are rushed or inexperienced. Angina and heart attack are commonly misdiagnosed in offices and emergency rooms, leading to tragic consequences.

What can you do to help avoid these costly treatment delays? Learn the unusual signs and symptoms of heart attack so you can quickly recognize if you or a loved one might be suffering from one. Most importantly, understand the reasons people themselves delay seeking emergency care when a heart attack strikes.

Risky Patient Delays in Seeking Care for a Heart Attack

Numerous studies have found some useful associations, trends and conclusions as to why people delay seeking treatment when angina or a heart attack strikes. The most basic reason people procrastinate is a lack of recognition that their symptoms are in fact those of a heart attack. One study found that central chest pain traveling to the arm or shoulder and collapse were the most common symptoms patients expected with a heart attack. More than half of the patients who suffered a heart attack felt actual symptoms that were very different than their expectations. Shortness of breath, excessive sweating, indigestion, back pain, and fatigue are common symptoms that heart attack sufferers experience, but may not identify as heart related.

Many psychological factors come into play during a heart attack. Some people may fear the emergency room or hospital and first seek treatment at a doctor's office or urgent care facility, wasting valuable time before getting definitive treatment with angioplasty or clot-dissolving medication. Some people simply delay seeking treatment because they don't want to admit they have a problem. Even those who know something is seriously wrong may fear death or disability and avoid seeking treatment.

Symptoms of a Heart Attack

The textbook symptoms of angina or a heart attack are a sudden pressing or constricting sensation in the chest beneath the breastbone, shortness of breath, pounding heart, sudden drenching sweat, nausea, vomiting or diarrhea, dizziness or passing out. New onset of tiring easily and becoming winded from walking up a hill or stairs can be a sign of heart disease. Chest pain that comes on with walking or activity and goes away with rest is more likely to be heart-related. The pressing sensation in the chest might travel to the neck, jaw or teeth, shoulders or arms (usually the left arm), back or even the abdomen. Any combination of the above symptoms can be present in someone with a heart problem. Some people experience *only* a toothache or shoulder pain or back pain or indigestion with belching during a heart attack. Diabetics are at higher risk for having no symptoms at all!

Your chest pain is *less* likely to be related to a heart problem when:

- Pain worsens with breathing or coughing.
- Pain increases with movement of your arms or torso, suggesting a rib or muscle injury.
- Pain increases by pressing on the ribs at the point where they meet the breastbone or sternum. Be wary of this finding since many people, particularly the elderly, will complain of pain when a doctor presses the ribs. This can mislead doctors into believing the problem is muscular.
- Pain is stabbing or sharp rather than "like someone is standing on my chest." This is also less reliable since people perceive and describe pain very differently. Adjectives commonly used by heart patients include squeezing, dull, ache, gas that won't come out, pressure and even sharp.
- The symptoms you feel now are exactly the same as when another problem was professionally diagnosed.

Physicians cannot easily distinguish symptoms of heart disease from other ailments. Do not trust any doctor who dismisses your chest pain complaint without considering and excluding more serious problems. If your chest pain symptoms last for five to fifteen minutes, cause breathing difficulty, dizziness, racing heart, recur over several days or worsen with walking or exertion then you must call your family doctor or seek medical help. If you have a past history of heart disease, call your doctor immediately if you experience chest pains or unfamiliar indigestion.

Chest Pain in Older Adults:
Special Considerations

Heart disease is the number one cause of death in older adults. People over age sixty-five are also at greater risk for complications and death from heart attack so early diagnosis and treatment are crucial. Identifying a heart attack in older adults, however, can be tricky for both patients and doctors, resulting in inadequate or improper treatment.

Heart attacks in older adults are more likely to show less typical features or to be "silent," without any symptoms. Chest pain is less likely as a symptom of heart attack in older adults, while shortness of breath is more common. Some proposed explanations why this age group tends to have less chest pain include decreased sensitivity to pain with aging, diminished ability to verbalize symptoms in some older adults and higher prevalence of diabetes, which predisposes to "silent" heart attacks.

It is not only the lack of chest pain that can make heart attack a difficult diagnosis in older adults. Vague symptoms such as weakness, fatigue, diminished ability to perform usual or daily activities, confusion, nausea and fainting are all possible presenting problems with heart attacks in this age group. Furthermore, heart attacks in this age group are less likely to show obvious electrocardiogram changes.

These difficulties in diagnosing heart attacks in older adults can result in misdiagnosis and improper treatment. Studies have shown that older patients are less likely to get treated with angioplasty, clot-dissolving drugs, and heart bypass surgery compared with younger patients. Since the elderly are more likely to have near-fatal heart attacks they might benefit most from these aggressive treatments. Rushed or inexperienced doctors can easily miss a heart attack or angina, a warning sign of serious heart disease, in older patients.

Older adults must learn about their risk factors for heart disease and the less typical manifestations of a heart attack or angina. If they seek care quickly and voice their concerns about having a heart attack, doctors will be less likely to miss a heart attack and more likely to treat it appropriately. The end result will be lives saved and less suffering.

Other Causes of Chest Pain

Two other potentially fatal causes of chest pain deserve mention, because doctors frequently overlook them: aortic dissection and pulmonary embolism. Misdiagnosis is more likely to occur with less typical symptoms of the illness, with inexperienced doctors, and if the diagnosis is simply not considered by the treating healthcare provider, an all too common occurrence with uncommon illness.

Aortic Dissection

Aortic dissection is a catastrophic illness that results from a tearing of the inner lining of the major body-feeding artery, the aorta, as it branches up from the heart. Blood then leaks into the space between layers of the artery lining causing a ballooning effect. Rupture or continued ballooning through the aorta can cause death. Less than half the patients who have this catastrophic illness are diagnosed before death, testimony to the difficulty diagnosing this serious complication.

Ninety-five percent of patients with this disorder will complain of mid-chest pain that begins abruptly and feels like "tearing" or "ripping" or "splitting" or "excruciating." Back pain is not uncommon. Shortness of breath and passing out can occur and some people might notice pain getting worse with each heartbeat. Chest X ray, CAT scan and echocardiogram can be helpful in confirming the diagnosis.

Pulmonary Embolism

The majority of clots that are "thrown" to the lungs come from a blood clot that forms in a deep leg vein. Common symptoms are difficulty breathing and chest pain that gets worse with a deep breath. Other signs or symptoms can include rapid breathing, racing heart, cough and leg swelling.

Risk factors for blood clots are being bedridden or sedentary, recent surgery, cancer, having a clot in the past, pregnancy, certain medications and heart problems. Tests that can help make the diagnosis include electrocardiogram, arterial blood gas, ventilation-perfusion scan, CAT scan and MRI.

STROKE

Stroke is the third leading cause of death in the United States and is also a leading cause of long-term disability in American adults. About one-third of stroke victims die within one year, and the death rate rises with increasing age. Clearly prevention is crucial yet many older adults—those who are at greatest risk for stroke—are less knowledgeable about symptoms of stroke than those of a heart attack.

Stroke has recently been declared a "brain attack" to remove this devastating illness from the "nothing-to-do-for-it" list and to treat it as aggressively as a heart attack. Time-dependent clot-dissolving treatment is available for eligible stroke sufferers within the first three hours after symptom onset. Even those who do not receive clot-dissolving treatment can benefit from earlier diagnosis and treatment, perhaps salvaging more brain cells and limiting disability.

There are two basic types of stroke during which nutrient-rich blood is cut off from a part of the brain, starving those cells and causing brain swelling, injury and cell death. About eighty percent of strokes are caused by a blood clot in a brain-feeding artery (ischemic). Clots can form within the artery itself from hardening of arteries and cholesterol plaque or a clot can be thrown into the blood system (embolism) and land in the brain. Embolic strokes most often arise because of heart conditions such as atrial fibrillation (irregular, disjointed beating and rhythm of the small heart chambers) and artificial or damaged heart valves.

A second common type of stroke comprises about twenty percent of the total—a brain bleed. Bleeding into the brain usually results from either longstanding high blood pressure, an aneurysm (ballooning) of a brain artery or a blood vessel abnormality called AVM. Bleeding into the brain causes swelling and inflammation, leading to the demise of brain cells.

These two varieties of stroke require very different treatment. A clot can be treated with either clot-dissolving medication or blood thinners. Controlling unusually high blood pressure can perhaps limit damage from a brain bleed. A CAT scan or MRI will diagnose a stroke and make this important diagnostic distinction. MRI has proven to be highly useful for diagnosing specific stroke types.

Symptoms of a Stroke

Stroke symptoms, similar to those of a heart attack, can be either dramatic or subtle. The types of symptoms depend upon the part of the brain that is affected. Symptoms and signs can include any combination of the following.
• Severe headache
• Seizure or coma
• Paralyzed or weak limb(s) on one side of the body
• Tingling or numbness in arm and/or leg and/or face
• Drooping corner of mouth
• Speech difficulties
• Nausea or vomiting
• Any change in mental function
• Blurred, dimmed or loss of vision
• Tingling or numbness around mouth, cheeks or gums
• Dizziness
• Sudden unexplained fall

Risk Factors for Stroke

Every year approximately 750,000 Americans and huge numbers worldwide suffer strokes and most of these people have more than one risk factor. Older adults are at greatest risk, particularly for "silent strokes" that cause no symptoms, but contribute to mental impairment.

Smoking cigarettes and high blood pressure are major risk factors predisposing to "silent" (lacunar) strokes. Despite older age being a major risk factor, nearly one-third of strokes strike people below age sixty-five.

Risks include:

1. Older age—the most powerful risk factor.
2. **Transient Ischemic Attack (TIA)** also known as "mini-stroke." Symptoms can include vision loss like a shade pulled over one eye; limb weakness, tingling or numbness; garbled speech; dizziness; headache; or swallowing difficulty. TIA is a key warning sign for stroke (and heart attack)! Five percent of people who suffer a TIA develop a full-blown stroke within one month, while one-third of TIA sufferers develop a stroke within five years.
3. Family history/genetics.
4. Ethnicity/minorities—African Americans, Hispanics and Native Americans have a higher risk of stroke than whites. African Americans between the ages of forty-five and sixty-four are four times more likely than whites to die from stroke.
5. High blood pressure, although modifiable, is a strong risk factor.
6. Diabetes mellitus is a significant risk factor.
7. Smoking one pack of cigarettes per day multiplies stroke risk by a factor of 2.5. Taking birth control pills concomitantly magnifies the risk. Quitting smoking reduces the risk.
8. Being overweight, especially obesity centered around the abdomen.
9. Plaque build-up in the neck (carotid) arteries poses a significant risk.
10. Atrial fibrillation, a disorganized and irregular beating of the smaller heart chambers, is the strongest heart-related risk factor for stroke, posing a six-fold increase in risk. Ten percent of adults over age seventy suffer from atrial fibrillation.
11. Being sedentary.
12. Deficiencies of vitamins B6, B12 or folic acid have been linked to increased risk for heart disease and stroke.
13. High blood levels of cholesterol increases stroke risk, but this association is less well defined than the cholesterol-heart attack connection.
14. Heavy alcohol use (moderate use—one to seven drinks per week—lowers stroke risk).
15. Illicit drug use such as cocaine, amphetamines and body building steroids are risk factors for stroke in younger adults.

16. Certain medical conditions increase stroke risk, such as sickle cell anemia, migraine headaches, sleep apnea and pregnancy. Heart disease and stroke also are closely linked for many reasons, including common underlying causes and throwing clots from the heart to the brain.

Those who have risk factors are urged to reduce their susceptibility by modifying risky behaviors, such as exercising more, making dietary changes, quitting smoking and drinking alcohol in moderation. A daily low dose aspirin can reduce chances for stroke in those at higher risk. Medical conditions such as diabetes and high blood pressure also should be carefully controlled.

Treatment Delays in Stroke

Unfortunately, the majority of people who suffer a stroke and who would benefit from clot-dissolving treatment often cannot get it because of delays beyond the three hour limit from symptom onset. Experts have rallied for establishing "stroke centers" in hospitals. These centers, if established, would be staffed by teams of stroke care experts who could rapidly diagnose and treat stroke victims.

Several factors contribute to delays in treating stroke sufferers. Stroke victims may not be able to call for help because of paralysis or speech difficulties. Those who live alone are at a disadvantage, because when a companion recognizes stroke symptoms chances are greater the victim will receive treatment more rapidly. Those who do not use 911 for transport are at greater risk for treatment delay. People who seek care at a doctor's office for symptoms highly suggestive of stroke, in an attempt to "avoid the hospital," are wasting precious time since they will wind up at an emergency room anyway. While in the ER, difficulty getting a CAT scan done also can contribute to treatment delay. When a doctor does not quickly recognize the subtle symptoms or signs of stroke or chooses not to treat stroke emergently as a "brain attack," costly treatment delays will occur.

The effectiveness of clot-dissolving treatment (tPA) for stroke is not as clear-cut as using this treatment for heart attack. Only one quality study to date has shown improvement in function (but no significant change in death rate) for those stroke patients treated with the clot-dissolving drug tissue plasminogen activator (tPA). Should someone who suffers what appears to be a relatively small stroke accept the risks of clot-dissolving therapy? These patients might choose to think long and hard (as long as it is less than three hours) before undergoing risky clot-dissolving therapy until scientists clarify this issue. Someone who suffers a massive or severe stroke, on the other hand, has far more to gain from clot-dissolving therapy.

Clot-dissolving therapy must be administered within **three hours** after symptom onset or benefits no longer outweigh risks. And the risks are quite significant. A brain bleed occurs as a complication of stroke *treatment* with tPA in over six percent of patients compared with about one percent of heart attack patients. Once again, the best medicine is prevention. People should learn about their risk factors for stroke and eliminate those that can be modified. Knowing all subtle and obvious symptoms and signs of stroke can help speed time to treatment.

USEFUL WEB SITES FOR STROKE INFORMATION

http://www.americanheart.org/warning.html#stroke
(Warning signs of stroke from the American Heart Association.)
http://www.stroke.org
(National Stroke Association's Web site.)
http://www.strokecenter.org
http://www.strokeassociation.org
(American Stroke Association.)
http://www.ninds.nih.gov
(National Institute of Neurological Disorders and Stroke's Web site.)
http://www.strokenetwork.org
(Stroke Support Network's Web site.)

SHORTNESS OF BREATH

Air hunger strikes a chord of panic even in the most stoic person. Shortness of breath can be caused by many heart or lung problems or can be a perception due to severe pain or anxiety. More common causes for breathing trouble are heart attack, heart failure, emphysema, asthma and hyperventilation. Fortunately, several telltale signs exist which suggest that a person's breathing difficulty can be serious and requires immediate medical attention:

- *Color:* If the person has a bluish tinge to their skin, lips, tongue or fingertips take it seriously.
- *Breathing Rate:* When the body is not getting enough oxygen the brain speeds up the breathing rate to suck in more air. Count the number of breaths the person is taking while timing thirty seconds on your watch. Multiply the number of breaths by two. The average breathing rate for adults is about fifteen breaths each minute;

the normal rate can be as high as sixty breaths each minute for newborns and thirty breaths each minute for a one-year old child. Harmless causes for a faster breathing rate include:
- Hyperventilation due to anxiety or pain
- Fever
- Normal individual variation (common in babies and toddlers)

- *Nasal Flaring:* Look at the nostrils. They can tell a great deal about a person's breathing, especially in a young child. If the nostrils widen then contract as if the person just ran a one hundred yard dash, then trouble might be brewing.

- *Accessory Breathing Muscles:* As the sick person breathes, look at the muscles in the neck where the shoulder meets the neck. These muscles normally cannot be seen contracting except when a person is oxygen-starved. The same is true of the intercostal muscles located between ribs. If you see fluttering between ribs, like a heartbeat under the skin, it is because these accessory muscles of breathing have kicked into action to help suck in needed air.

- *Wheezing and Bubbling:* Put your ear against the person's back and ask the sick person to take a deep breath in and out through the mouth. If you hear wheezing sounds it might be an asthma attack. Crackling and bubbling sounds suggest either infection or water in the lungs and the person's appearance and other symptoms will determine what to do. Does the ill person have any other signs of breathing compromise? If so, call an ambulance. If not, call your doctor.

- *Sitting Forward/Not Lying Flat:* People suffering from an attack of asthma or emphysema will usually sit upright, arms propping their body forward. A person suffering from heart failure with water backed up in the lungs may not be able to sleep flat on the back.

- *Leg Swelling:* Swelling in both ankles that leaves a finger impression from pressure can be a clue to heart failure.

- *Talking or Silent:* If the person can barely utter a sentence, call 911 immediately! If the person complains of shortness of breath, but is having a full conversation with you, you probably have some time to call a doctor for advice.

ABDOMINAL PAIN

You are hunched over with stabbing pain in your belly. Is it just gas from the chili you ate last night? A stomach virus? Appendicitis?

Believe it or not, up to forty percent of patients with abdominal pain will leave the emergency room without a sure answer. It is difficult for physicians to identify the cause of abdominal or pelvic pain, even after performing tests. So do not try your luck at self-diagnosis.

Bear in mind, there are no simple tests that easily diagnose the cause for an abdominal illness such as appendicitis. A special type of CAT scan can help to pinpoint a diagnosis. The only sure way to diagnose appendicitis is to operate and look inside the abdomen. A medical history, physical examination, basic laboratory tests and specialized testing like CAT scan or ultrasound can provide clues to help arrive at a diagnosis.

Pain in the abdomen is the major complaint in six to eight percent of ER visits and two to four percent of doctors' office visits each year. Oftentimes, no definite answer is found, but the pain will resolve with simple dietary measures, simple medications and time. Close follow-up within twelve to twenty-four hours is prudent for all but the most mild and trivial abdominal complaints in which a confident diagnosis has not been reached. Belly pain may seem trivial early in the evolution of serious medical and surgical emergencies. The serious causes, however, will progress over hours to unbearable or life-threatening illness, while more benign causes for abdominal pain will become intermittent or improve. A few hours of intravenous fluids and observation in the office or emergency room does wonders for distinguishing serious from benign causes for abdominal pain. Most patients will improve after two large bags of salt water, some time, reassurance and simple remedies while awaiting basic test results.

Further Clues to Serious Causes of Abdominal or Pelvic Pain

The only rule with abdominal pain is there are no rules. Several clues, however, point to a more serious reason for abdominal pain. Often, these guidelines are far less reliable in infants and the elderly.

Fever: Fever between 99.5 and 101 degrees Fahrenheit is more typical of appendicitis, while temperatures in the range of 102 to 104 degrees Fahrenheit make abdominal, pelvic, or kidney infection more likely. Any fever with abdominal pain, however, should give you more cause for concern.

Progression of Pain: Pain that comes on strong and suddenly then remains severe or quickly becomes unbearable is ominous. Mild pain that does not go away and gradually gets worse over a few hours is also concerning. In such cases, using simple measures like taking Tylenol or an antacid are unlikely to help much.

Bleeding: Blood comes in several varieties including red, maroon to purple, or black (called coffee ground in vomit, melena in feces). If you see any of these forms of blood seek medical advice or attention.

Advanced Age: Like oil and vinegar, older age and belly pain do not mix. Abdominal pain in an older person is more likely to be serious. Studies have shown about one-third of older adults who go to an emergency room with abdominal pain will end up having surgery.

Medication Use: People who take prednisone or aspirin-like medication are at greater risk for serious abdominal ailments. Ask your doctor about your medications or research them in the *Physician's Desk Reference* or product information sheet. Any medication can cause abdominal pains but some are more commonly associated with pain in the abdomen, so check the listed side effects of your medications.

Rapid Heartbeat: Measure your pulse while you are in good health so you have a baseline value. If you then measure your pulse rate while experiencing belly pain, it will be easier to know if it is truly rapid for *you*. If your temperature is normal, a pulse rate above one hundred to one hundred ten beats per minute (average being sixty to eighty) is more concerning. If your pulse is normally forty-eight then a heart rate of ninety beats per minute might be considered rapid for you, near normal for others. Fever itself increases the heart rate about ten beats per minute for each one degree of Fahrenheit temperature elevation. Without fever, however, a rapid heartbeat might be a clue to dehydration or serious infection.

Activities of Daily Living: Those who suffer from a life-threatening cause of abdominal pain will *not* be able to continue the usual activities of the day, with the rare exception of a few stoic people with a high pain threshold. A nagging stomach ulcer, on the other hand, *is* serious but is not usually life-threatening. An ulcer sufferer perhaps will be able to take an over-the-counter remedy and resume daily activities.

Patient Position: If the sick individual is lying still and does not want to move that is more ominous. Someone who is lying still with knees bent up closer to the chest (curled or fetal position) is more likely to have serious inflammation in the abdomen. A person who writhes on the bed or circles around the room searching for, but not finding, a comfortable position might, for instance, have the colicky pain of a kidney stone or intestinal ailment.

Pain Quality and Location: Pain that originates from an abdominal organ is often more serious. We have all experienced a more benign example of this type of pain: cramping intestinal pain caused by food poisoning or burning pain from a mild stomach ulcer. Serious causes for pain originating from an organ in the belly (called visceral pain) include appendicitis, gallbladder attack or severe intestinal or other organ disease. This type of pain is felt as dull, cramping or burning. It is gradual in onset and vague, being felt somewhere in the midline of the abdomen along a vertical line drawn from the breast bone down through the belly button to the groin. Visceral pain usually is accompanied by sweats, nausea or vomiting. Interestingly, organs themselves have no sensation. Only tension or stretching of the *lining* of organs causes pain. If blood flow to an organ is cut off that organ will begin to die, causing visceral pain. When a nerve inside the abdomen is irritated from inflammation or a tumor it will cause pain. Inflammation of the thin membranes lining the abdominal and pelvic cavities will cause a sharper, more intense, and easily pinpointed type of pain. This "somatic" pain is what causes the movement of pain to the lower right abdomen during an appendix attack, for instance. Pain located only in the right, upper part of the abdomen is more likely to be from gallbladder or liver problems when the abdominal lining gets inflamed in that location. Pain localized in the lower abdomen or pelvis can be a gynecologic problem in women or testicular problem in men.

Nausea, Vomiting, Loss of Appetite: If you throw up more than once, your abdominal pain is more concerning. If your ailment proves to be just a stomach virus or food poisoning, vomiting puts you at greater risk for dehydration. Persistent vomiting is particularly worrisome in infants, the elderly and diabetics.

Female Problems: Belly or pelvic pain with unusual vaginal discharge or bleeding (not related to menstruation) requires prompt medical attention. Painful intercourse can be a sign of pelvic inflammatory disease (PID), a potentially serious infection.

Male Problems: Ailments of the testicles or hernias can cause lower abdominal pain. Be particularly cautious in males under age twenty-five because they are more likely to have a twisted testicle (torsion) causing abdominal pain. Many doctors overlook testicular problems in males who have belly pain. What's more, many male patients are too embarrassed to admit they are experiencing pain in the genitals.

Heart Disease: Those who have heart problems or major risk factors for heart disease such as high blood pressure, diabetes, family members with heart attacks, high cholesterol or smoking should take abdominal pain seriously. Heart attacks often cause upper abdominal and not chest pain.

Commonly Misdiagnosed
Abdominal Emergencies

There are several abdominal emergencies that deserve special mention because they are frequently misdiagnosed or overlooked, the consequences of which can be deadly.

Appendicitis

Since about eight out of every one hundred people will develop appendicitis in their lifetime, with its life-threatening potential, prompt diagnosis is crucial to prevent rupture and its complications. The most *typical* symptoms of appendicitis are sudden onset of vague abdominal pain *first,* usually around or above the belly button, followed by loss of appetite, nausea, or vomiting. Low grade fever can develop next. A sharper and more severe pain soon appears in the right lower abdomen when the lining of the abdomen in that area becomes inflamed (somatic pain). Constipation is much more common than diarrhea.

As serious as it may be, appendicitis is commonly misdiagnosed. Just because you are experiencing pain in the right lower abdomen does not mean you have appendicitis. To further confuse the diagnosis, just because your pain is *not* in the lower right abdomen it is no guarantee you do *not* have appendicitis.

Someone suffering from lower abdominal pain who seeks care at an emergency room might get one of four treatment approaches. If the ER doctor believes appendicitis is highly likely, a surgeon will evaluate the patient and operate immediately if the surgeon concurs. A second approach can be overnight hospitalization if appendicitis is strongly suspected, but the diagnosis is in doubt and the patient is clearly very ill. If the patient's illness progresses despite intravenous fluids and time, the surgeon will operate. A third treatment approach might be several hours of emergency department observation, intravenous fluids and simple remedies if the ER doctor is uncertain of the diagnosis. The last approach will be a few basic diagnostic tests and then being sent home. Nowadays, a helical CAT scan more than likely will be performed for ill patients in whom the diagnosis is uncertain.

So you suddenly develop pain in the lower right side of the abdomen. Is it appendicitis? Because appendicitis is quite common and potentially deadly if treatment is delayed, this diagnosis must always be considered in any person who is having abdominal pain. If appendicitis is missed and it ruptures, it can lead to overwhelming infection, pus pockets forming in the abdominal cavity, part of the intestines dying and even patient death.

Key Appendicitis Facts And Clues

- Appendicitis probably has more exceptions than rules so never dismiss it as a diagnosis. Pain in the pelvis or upper, right part of the abdomen are possible areas of pain with appendicitis. Pain does not have to be in the lower right part of the abdomen. In rare cases, some people have their appendix on the *left* side!
- When pain begins around the belly button and soon shifts to the lower right part of the abdomen, the diagnosis should be appendicitis until proven otherwise.
- An inflamed appendix will usually perforate (burst open) within forty-eight hours.
- The pain caused by a diseased abdominal organ can be mild at onset, but it builds steadily without any relief.
- People suffering from serious abdominal or pelvic disease will often remain still on their side in a curled position, bent at the waist, and with their knees pulled in close to their chests. Coughing aggravates the pain as does riding over bumps in the car.
- Fevers above 102 degrees Fahrenheit suggest a diagnosis *other than* appendicitis.
- Fever can be absent with appendicitis.
- When a blood count (CBC) and abdominal X ray are normal, they *do not* rule out appendicitis.
- Nausea or vomiting is present in only two-thirds to three-quarters of patients suffering from appendicitis. Loss of appetite is, however, almost always present.
- It is not uncommon for people with appendicitis to have urinary symptoms and even a mildly abnormal urine test. Do not let a doctor jump to the conclusion of a mild urinary tract infection if you feel quite ill.

Appendicitis Tips

1. Ask your treating doctor if he or she is confident your abdominal pain is *not* serious. Does the doctor have a clear-cut diagnosis that is consistent with your symptoms? You are not likely to have a mild urinary tract infection, for instance, if you are having the worst abdominal pain of your life or if you have had urinary infections before and this illness is far worse.
2. Any responsible doctor will reevaluate a patient having bad abdominal pain and an uncertain diagnosis. Re-evaluation should be done within six to twelve hours maximum, not a couple of days.

3. It is not prudent to accept phone advice from a doctor regarding abdominal pain. If your doctor does not feel it is important to examine you for unfamiliar abdominal pain, you are probably better off getting another doctor.
4. A helical CAT scan can be very helpful if a doctor or surgeon suspects, yet is unsure, about appendicitis. Do not go under the knife without a CAT scan unless your doctor is confident it is appendicitis or if you are so ill that surgery cannot be delayed.
5. Three simple tests anyone can do can be helpful in distinguishing serious causes for abdominal pain.
   a. Heel-drop jarring test: Stand on your toes for fifteen seconds then come down with all your weight on the heels. If this causes pain in the lower abdomen it is more likely to be serious.
   b. Cough test: If coughing aggravates pain in the lower abdomen it is more concerning.
   c. Hopping on one foot: If someone with abdominal pain can easily hop on one foot without much problem, the cause for abdominal pain is *less* likely to be appendicitis or an inflammation of the inside lining of the abdomen.

Appendicitis In Older Adults

About five percent of abdominal emergencies in older adults prove to be appendicitis and this diagnosis is frequently missed. In fact, one-third of older adults who are hospitalized for abdominal pain will undergo exploratory surgery. Abdominal pain is more easily misdiagnosed and more likely to be serious in this age group for a variety of reasons, including other illnesses and medications that can confuse the diagnostic picture, a lessening of tenderness and lack of abdominal wall muscle tensing in the older patient and, frequently, delay in seeking treatment.

One additional type of abdominal medical crisis in older adults deserves mention because it is also commonly overlooked. When blood supply to organs in the abdomen is cut off from a blood clot, aneurysm (ballooning), or other causes, the result is that nutrient-starved organs begin to die, particularly the intestines. These emergencies typically cause severe cramping or burning pain yet the abdominal examination seems relatively normal. That is the most important clue in combination with risk factors for blood vessel (vascular) abdominal emergencies. Risks include recent heart attack, history of heart disease, atrial fibrillation, heart failure, prior blood clot, and others. If this abdominal emergency is overlooked, the person will quickly deteriorate and die as abdominal organs starve to death from lack of blood supply.

FRACTURES

A fracture is an interruption or break in the normal structure of a bone. Contrary to popular belief, most fractures do *not* require any special treatment and heal themselves in time. Examples of common, self-healing fractures include simple breaks of the nose, fingers, toes and ribs.

Another common misconception is that, "I thought if it was broken, I wouldn't be able to move it." This is simply not true. Pain may persuade a person to keep the injured body part still. Swelling often causes stiffness near a joint. Fear of making it worse typically makes movement of the injured part difficult as well. In fact, if the injured part truly *cannot* be moved, that would be a sign of a serious injury that requires immediate attention. Other clues pointing to a more serious injury include: the injured part appearing deformed; a lot of swelling (which can also make it appear deformed); bluish, pale, or mottled discoloration of skin; numbness or pins and needles; an open wound above the injured area which can lead to a bone infection; a break in a bone that extends into a joint; and a high-risk injury such as high-speed car accident or fall from a roof or severe crush injuries.

Most growth plate injuries in children are minor and heal fine without complications. However, injury to the line across bones at which growth continues to occur in children can occasionally cause complications, requiring early diagnosis and proper expert treatment.

Common Types Of Fractures

- *Avulsion* – the rubber band-like supporting ligament tears off a small bone fragment.
- *Displaced* – when the edge of the injured bone moves out of its normal location. These commonly occur in wrist fractures, for instance, and require realigning the bone edges. Surgery is not necessarily required for this.
- *Open* – open wound that extends directly to the broken bone.
- *Pathologic* – a break in a previously weakened bone due to another bone disease such as osteoporosis or cancer.
- *Stress* – stress fracture is a thin line of weakened bone resulting from excessive stress on that bone. Commonly occurs in foot and leg bones among joggers, for instance.

- *Unstable* — a fracture with odd shaped or oblique edges that will not stay in place with a cast. These usually require an operation to secure the fragments or edges with plates or screws.

Tips on Fractures

- For comfort, the injured area should be splinted before the patient is sent for an X ray in the ER. Pain medicine should also be given, but is often neglected. Patients or family must *ask* for pain medicine.
- The majority of fractures do *not* require treatment by an orthopedist.
- Two key things doctors check for with any injury is that enough blood is getting past the injured site and that there is no nerve damage. Tingling or pins and needles can be a sign of nerve damage. Bluish, pale or mottled skin discoloration or loss of a pulse are signs blood flow has been compromised. This can lead to tissue death and loss of limb.
- Not every fracture requires a full cast. Many heal fine with just a splint. A full cast may not be applied right away even if needed because as swelling increases over the first two to three days, a cast can become uncomfortable or even lead to complications.
- Certain types of fractures have a greater risk for complications such as a "navicular (scaphoid)" fracture of the wrist, "supracondylar" fracture of the elbow (common with falls from monkey bars), and "Jones" fracture of the foot, to name just a few. These should be referred for treatment by an orthopedist. If future function is at risk, as might be the case with hand fractures in a musician or leg injuries in an athlete, for example, a specialist should be consulted.
- Treatment of an injury with swelling should include "**RICE**": Rest, Ice packs (not ice directly on skin), Compression with a tape wrap or ace bandage and Elevation to reduce swelling. Pain medication is also appropriate, if needed.

LACERATIONS

Your body is working to stop the bleeding even before the palm of your hand presses down on that gushing gash. Torn blood vessels narrow, blood coagulates and platelets clump to plug the hole. Indeed, most cuts stop bleeding and heal on their own.

Why then should people seek medical care when that knife slips or razor slashes? Your amazing body sometimes needs a helping hand. When your palm applies direct pressure over the wound, most cuts will stop bleeding within fifteen to thirty minutes. Potential complications, however, are the primary reason to seek professional care.

Bleeding

If bleeding does not stop after thirty minutes of firm pressure directly over the cut or if you see blood spurting into the air like a water fountain, you might have cut a larger vein or artery. Taking blood thinners such as aspirin or coumadin can also lead to prolonged bleeding. Keep pressing down firmly over the wound while you seek medical care.

Infection

Any break in the skin allows bacteria into the wound and that poses a risk for infection. Contaminants that pose the greatest risk for infection include soil, gravel, saliva, feces, plant matter and any wood, glass or metal objects. The longer the delay in having a wound cleaned and stitched, the greater chance for infection. Lacerations should be treated within about six hours or risk for infection rises quickly. Cuts on the face and scalp can safely be cleaned and closed within twelve to twenty-four hours after injury. Any wound that needs stitching for cosmetic reasons such as a facial laceration should be stitched even after the usual twenty-four hour limit.

What do you do when the blood starts to gush? Apply direct pressure first for brisk bleeding. Elevate the bleeding body part. When bleeding slows or stops, rinse the wound with soap and water or watered down povidone/iodine solution. Bacitracin ointment and a dressing or bandage complete the first aid treatment.

If you have not had a tetanus booster within five years, you should get one for wounds which are deep; more than six hours old; contaminated with soil, gravel or other foreign material; or infected. Star-like cuts, crush cuts, and cuts in which a chunk of skin is sliced or gouged off require having had a tetanus shot within the previous five years. Clean, simple cuts less than six hours old and not infected require tetanus immunization within the past ten years.

Hidden Damage from Wounds

Wounds can be deceiving. Tin can lids can slice hand tendons and nerves in a wound that resembles a paper cut. Motorized and power tools tend to do more damage deep inside the flesh. A major reason to seek experienced medical care is to detect hidden damage in a cut, whether the wound appears minor or is obviously severe.

Hand lacerations pose the greatest risk for hidden damage since many nerves and tendons are packed into a small space. Deep cuts must be checked carefully since a sliced tendon can cause loss of function. If you are unable to fully bend or straighten fingers, a tendon is probably severed. Loss of strength with finger bending or straightening can also be a clue to hidden damage. If you can see a glistening white band (a tendon) at the base of the cut, hidden damage is more likely. Complete loss of feeling on one side of a finger beyond the cut indicates a nerve was sliced. A hand surgeon should reattach the nerve. The only way to carefully check for hidden damage is for an experienced doctor to stop the bleeding then examine the wound, usually after injection of numbing medication. Small cuts to fingertips that do not involve the nail bed (underneath the nail) are not likely to be serious.

Cuts to the nail beds, the pink skin just beneath fingernails, can heal with scarring deformity if not treated properly. Only physicians experienced in repairing these cuts should handle nail bed lacerations.

Facial lacerations can cause damage to nerve or muscle and should get expert repair as well. Cuts close to the eyes or involving the eyelids can have hidden damage to important muscles or tear ducts. These require expert repair by a plastic surgeon or ophthalmologist.

Facial Wounds

Cuts on the face present a whole new set of rules. The face has many landmarks, borders, and creases that contribute to your appearance. These borders and creases might be permanently changed if lacerations are not repaired properly. This is particularly true of cuts near eyes, on lips and on earlobes. Jagged cuts are far more complex than straight, clean wounds. Vertical (from forehead toward chin) face cuts go against normal skin creases and might require a surgeon's expertise for the best outcome. Request a plastic surgeon when in doubt.

Do I Need Immediate Medical Care for My Cut? Where Should I Go?

Ask yourself the following questions to decide if you must seek medical attention for a laceration.

1. *How Did I Cut Myself?* Injuries from power tools, tin-can lids, glass and car accidents are more likely to result in hidden damage or complications. Is a tendon or nerve sliced deep inside? Might there be a piece of metal, wood, glass or gravel inside the wound?

2. *Is Bleeding Persistent?* You've applied direct pressure for twenty to thirty minutes and it continues to bleed or blood spurts like a fountain if you release pressure. Get medical attention.

3. *Location: Where Is the Cut?* Cuts to the hands, face, lips, area around the eye and beneath fingernails are more likely to cause complications in function or appearance. These wounds are more likely to require repair by a surgeon, not a primary care physician.

4. *Appearance: What Does It Look Like?* Is there a gap between skin edges? Is a hand laceration more than half an inch long? Is the cut jagged, star-shaped or dirty? Is yellow fat protruding outside the wound? Can you see a glistening, white tendon at the base of the wound? Yes to these questions suggests you should get medical attention.

5. *Miscellaneous:* Am I diabetic? Was my cut from an animal or human bite? Am I taking medication such as prednisone or chemotherapy that can delay healing? Is my immune system seriously weakened from cancer, kidney failure, AIDS or other serious chronic disease? Do I have a heart valve problem that might need preventive antibiotic treatment? If you've answered yes to any of these questions, seek medical care.

Once you have decided to get medical attention for your laceration, your choice of facility depends in part on the time of day. During office hours, try to go directly to a plastic or hand surgeon for high-risk face or hand cuts. Call your family doctor if you need a referral. If you belong to an HMO, you might have to first see your primary care doctor before going to a specialist.

A reputable urgent or immediate care office in your community is a good alternative to have simpler wounds evaluated. Be suspicious of any facility reluctant to refer you to a specialist for high-risk wounds on the hands or face. You should know that most primary care doctors (internists or pediatricians) do not stitch lacerations.

General Care and Advice for Lacerations

1. Avoid emergency rooms if possible. If you stop the bleeding from a cut sustained during early morning hours (after two A.M.), it is safe to gently clean it and wait a few hours more for office hours. Even for bad facial cuts, you can usually wait several hours to get treated at a plastic surgeon's office. Scalp cuts bleed a lot, but they can wait several hours to be sutured if you stop the bleeding.

2. If you choose to delay seeking care, stop the bleeding then gently clean the wound with soap and water or povidone/iodine solution in water. A reminder: Do not wait longer than several hours. Cuts should generally be treated as soon as possible to reduce risk for infection, particularly lacerations on the hand.
3. Teaching hospitals are perhaps the worst place to get treatment for lacerations! Cuts will probably be stitched by a medical student, Intern, Resident or physician assistant. Treatment might be competent or absolutely horrific depending on the experience (clue: watch how much his or her hands shake), skill and common sense of that caretaker.
4. At community hospitals, the Attending emergency physician is usually (not always) somewhat more experienced with lacerations. Because of time constraints, if the cut is high-risk (on the hands or face) or complex or if you request a specialist, the community hospital emergency doctor will gladly call in a plastic, hand or general surgeon to care for it.

HEAD PAIN

"I have a splitting headache" means different things to different people. Some headaches can be nagging yet not prevent a person from carrying on with normal activities. Other headaches can be debilitating, rendering a person bedridden in a dark, quiet room. Headaches can also be unbearable and potentially deadly! The most common types of headaches are:
• Muscle contraction (tension) headache
• Vascular headache (includes migraine and cluster types)

There are many other causes for headache pain including eye problems, high blood pressure, sinus problems, neck problems, dental or tooth problems, meningitis, brain aneurysm, inflammation of a scalp artery (temporal arteritis) and others. By the length of the list, it is clear that you should not serve as your own doctor. What you need to do is decide whether your head pain is potentially serious or not.

Tension headaches typically cause constant, band-like pain in the back of the head, neck or forehead areas. These headaches can generally last from thirty minutes to seven days. A key distinguishing feature from migraine headaches is that this type usually does *not* prevent the sufferer from continuing activities of daily living.

Migraine headaches cause throbbing pain often, but not exclusively, on one side of the head and may be accompanied by: nausea, vomiting, pain or eye-tearing from light exposure, over-sensitivity to noise and a need to be in a dark, quiet room. Severe pains generally last from four to seventy-two hours and can be intensified with normal activities such as stair climbing. Common triggers for migraine headache are caffeine, chocolate, menstruation, stress or exertion.

Cluster headaches cause stabbing, recurrent headaches on one side of the head and can be accompanied by eye redness or tearing, runny nose or congestion and sometimes a small pupil and droopy eyelid on the painful side. Cluster headache sufferers may have several short attacks daily (on average, sixty to ninety minutes each) and pace the floor because of severe pain.

Both tension and migraine headaches used to be considered as two clearly distinguishable entities, but we now know that is not the case. These headaches can share many features, making diagnosis difficult. Similar symptoms may also indicate a much more severe problem. There are several important questions to ask yourself that can help you decide if your headache is serious from causes such as brain aneurysm, high blood pressure/stroke or meningitis.

Questions to Ask Yourself about Head Pain

1. Have I ever had this type of headache at this intensity before? If you have, try simple pain remedies or an analgesic prescribed by your doctor. If this is your first headache ever and you are over age thirty-five then consult your physician. Most people with tension or migraine headaches have had them before age thirty-five.
2. Was the pain explosive at onset or is this by far the worst headache of my life? If so, immediately call your doctor or seek help.
3. Is the pain sudden and unbearable or has it slowly progressed and is more of a nuisance? A slowly developing headache that allows you to continue activity will probably respond to home pain relievers. A debilitating, unfamiliar headache that comes on suddenly requires a call to your doctor or a visit to an emergency care facility.
4. Is the headache accompanied by other symptoms such as fever, arm or leg weakness or numbness, confusion or difficulty with memory, distorted vision, lethargy or clumsiness? Did the severity of the headache awaken you from sleep? These instances suggest a more serious cause and require immediate medical attention.

5. Is the headache brought on by exertion? Is it accompanied by a stiff neck? Both harmless and serious problems can cause this so consult your doctor.
6. Did you suffer a head injury in the days or weeks before the headache began? Even if the head injury seemed minor, it might signal a more serious problem.
7. Do you have other medical conditions that might play a role in the headache such as high blood pressure, cancer or a weakened immune system? In this case, sudden or severe headache should cause you to consult with your physician.

HIGH FEVERS

Sir William Osler wrote: "Humanity has but three great enemies: Fever, famine and war. Of these, by far the greatest, by far the most terrible, is fever." Dr. Osler, a revered physician, spoke of fever as a sign of infection. His concerns were legitimate in a time when antibiotics to treat serious infections did not exist. Today, parents need not turn fever into such a hot issue. A rise in the body's temperature set point, or fever, is not a disease, but a warning sign of illness and the body's response in an effort to fight the disease.

Infection is not always the culprit for a rising body temperature. Some benign and common causes of fever are physical activity, a hot summer day (ambient temperature can raise body temperature), inaccurate use of or reading of the thermometer and normal daily temperature variation that is usually at its peak of about 100.3 degrees Fahrenheit between 6:00 P.M. and 10:00 P.M. Some people are normally on the high end, others normally on the low end of the temperature scale.

Should you be worried about fever? Fever itself is usually not a serious concern and only fevers greater than 106 degrees Fahrenheit risk causing brain damage. Fever is the body's natural and clever response to help fight disease. At higher body temperatures, infection-fighting white blood cells move faster and kill bacteria better. Fever shrinks the iron supply in blood, iron being a necessary ingredient for bacteria to survive.

Fever is not all good. Higher body temperatures above 101 degrees Fahrenheit are uncomfortable and cause lassitude and muscle wasting. More significantly, fever increases the work demand of the heart and lungs and that can tip a delicate balance in those who have heart or lung disease. A *rapid* rise in body temperature (more than how high the fever goes) can precipitate febrile seizures in susceptible children. People with epilepsy are at greater risk for suffering a seizure from high body temperature. The elderly often become confused and lethargic from high fever. Herpes simplex infections (fever blisters, cold sores) can be reactivated by fever as well. In addition, fever burns up more body fluid and can hasten dehydration. It is also possible, but not certain, that high fever can harm the fetus during the first three months of pregnancy.

When someone has a rising fever, they will experience shivering or chills. A red, flushed face can be a sign the fever has peaked, especially in children. Finally, a drenching sweat suggests the fever is breaking.

How do you best manage fever? Do not panic. Do not grab your coat and rush to the emergency room. Use the following simple measures to reduce fever. These measures might make the sick person (as well as family members) more comfortable:

- Keep the patient's room comfortably cool.
- Avoid excessive sweaters, blankets, and other clothing that prevent heat evaporation (which could raise body temperature).
- Bathing in lukewarm bath water might be helpful, but cool or cold sponging or bathing can be harmful. Cool water is uncomfortable to sit in and can cause shivering which increases body temperature. Cool water also causes blood vessels in the skin to narrow, trapping more heat in the body instead of heat evaporating away.
- Never use isopropyl rubbing alcohol to sponge someone with fever. The chemical is toxic.
- Give a sick person a household fever reducing remedy in the appropriate dosage. It will take at least forty-five minutes until fever begins to drop. Under dosing of fever-lowering remedies is a common cause for persistently high fever.
- Fever can produce strange symptoms and behavior. If a person's behavior or alertness does not return to normal after administering acetaminophen or ibuprofen to reduce the fever, seek medical care immediately.

PART

4

HOW TO AVOID
PEDIATRIC PERILS

It's a parent's worst nightmare. Suddenly baby's limbs flail in a seizure. Or your child turns blue and stares blankly. Or your toddler bangs his head and is so sleepy he can't look at you. You're frantic. Sheer panic clouds your thinking. *What should I do first? Should I call the pediatrician? Drive the baby to the nearest emergency room? Shake him until he responds?* Unfortunately, none of these responses may be correct.

Panic is a reflex reaction when your child falls ill or gets injured. Advance preparation can change the reflex arc from panic to productivity. What do you do if your baby turns blue or becomes drowsy and unresponsive? What if a child falls from a tree? Do you call your pediatrician? Probably not since there will not be time to wait for the return phone call. Drive baby to an emergency room? If you live within five minutes of a hospital, that is reasonable for serious illness. Severe injuries such as falling from a tree or being hit by a car should be managed by trained professionals. Moving a severely injured person without proper care can do irreversible harm to a serious neck injury, for instance. Since most people live more than seven minutes away from the nearest hospital, do not drive a seriously ill child to the hospital unless no ambulance is available. Lack of oxygen to the brain can do permanent damage in less than five minutes. Call for an ambulance since they can more quickly implement life support techniques and administer oxygen. Besides, you should not drive fast while in a cloud of panic.

Should a parent or caretaker shake a baby to get a response? Never! Shaking a baby can be harmful. Rub the child's cheek, chest or shoulder while calling his or her name. What someone should do at this point is taught in a Basic Life Support (BLS) course. Every parent and child caretaker should learn the basic skills to check for breathing and a pulse,. to reposition the airway (breathing) passage, to treat choking victims and to perform mouth-to-mouth breathing and cardiopulmonary resuscitation (CPR) until professional help arrives. For BLS course listings, check out the American Heart Association, American Red Cross, and other Web sites. In addition, there are Web sites that have step-by-step choking, mouth-to-mouth breathing and CPR instructions with illustrations (see page 173).

Writing out a last will and testament is unpleasant enough, but the task of anticipating serious illness or injury in your child is plainly repulsive. Most people would prefer to avoid thoughts of a child being stricken, but medical calamity does strike the nursery. People should not be passive when their children's health is at stake. It behooves parents to plan ahead and endure unpleasant thoughts so they might prevent suffering through tragic reality.

Consider these troubling statistics:

- There are over twenty million pediatric emergency room visits annually in this country.
- The death rate is higher for serious injury in children compared to similar injuries in adults. The increased death rate is magnified in areas without special pediatric care centers.
- Injuries claim about 10,000 children's lives each year, and are the leading cause of death and disability among children ages one to fourteen, according to the Center for Disease Control Mortality files.
- Thousands more children die each year from treatable illness such as asthma, meningitis and other bacterial infections.
- When children stop breathing, more than fifty percent of them can survive if prompt and proper care is given.
- Children under age three tend to put objects in their mouths, putting them at high risk for choking.
- Poisoning accounts for about 5000 deaths and eight million illnesses every year in this country. The majority of poisonings involve children below five years of age.

Do not get scared, get prepared! A sound, advance plan of action is crucial to avoid panic and mistakes at a moment of crisis. Many dangers threaten the health of our children: car accidents, poisoning, choking, drowning, firearm injuries, bicycle injuries, falls from heights or down stairs, burns and serious illness like asthma and meningitis. Surely the best medicine for our children is prevention. Sadly, another serious threat to the well-being of our children is our own emergency care system. Our nation's emergency care system is set up to care primarily for adults and not children.

What are the consequences of an emergency system that considers children as an afterthought? Countless children may die or become disabled from avoidable catastrophes. If you believe the ambulance technician or nurse or emergency doctor will do everything possible with skill and expertise to save your child's life, you are taking a lot for granted. Healthcare professionals save the lives of many kids. But many of these emergency workers are simply inadequately trained to care for very sick children.

Consider these distressing facts:

- An Institute of Medicine report on emergency medical services for children confirmed the inadequate pediatric training of ambulance technicians (EMTs) and paramedics.[1] According to the report, EMTs and paramedics spend only a few hours learning how to stabilize sick babies and young children, just a small fraction of their total training.

- In rural states, up to ninety percent of ambulance workers are volunteers who have virtually no pediatric care training. Furthermore, since most emergency care professionals do not often treat seriously ill babies, the emotional trauma of seeing a suffering child can worsen confusion and uneasiness during such a medical crisis.

- Nurses play a crucial role in all phases of emergency care, according to the IOM report, yet a survey found that ninety-five percent of nurses did not take the pediatric advanced life support course and did not receive specific pediatric care training from their hospital.

- The American Heart Association's revised advanced cardiac life support (ACLS) curriculum has little coverage of critical care for children. A large proportion of primary care physicians and nurses become certified in the ACLS course. Why then is pediatric care training at a minimum in this standard training course given to a majority of emergency healthcare workers?

- About fifteen percent of admissions to neonatal and pediatric intensive care units involved medication errors, according to one study.[2]

- Alarmingly, a study revealed that pediatric patients under age two

and those in the intensive care unit are at greatest risk for medication errors.[3]
• Dosage calculation errors are common in pediatrics. Some studies have shown that about one in twelve dosage calculations in a neonatal intensive care unit involved a ten-fold decimal.[4]

Several years back, a *U.S. News and World Report* article brought many key issues in pediatric emergency care to the public's attention.[5] The article summarized the findings of a pediatric emergency medical service report. "Every day, some of America's children die, or almost die, because they are taken to the wrong hospital, treated with improper equipment, given wrong dosages of medications or not diagnosed properly," the magazine article warned.

Our nation's emergency care system was designed for adults, not babies and young children. Few hospitals have separate pediatric emergency rooms that are staffed by pediatricians trained in emergency care. Those that do are mostly major teaching hospitals.

Babies and young children are at a distinct disadvantage in our emergency system from the moment the ambulance arrives all the way through their emergency room evaluation. Despite recent changes to improve EMT and paramedic training in pediatric care, one study found that a majority of emergency medical technicians and paramedics experienced great concern if called to care for a critically ill or injured child under age three. This may well be due in part to inadequate pediatric training and experience. When paramedics are called to care for a seriously ill or injured child, they infrequently perform stabilizing procedures such as inserting a breathing tube or intravenous line. These procedures are more difficult to perform on young children and paramedics (as well as nurses and doctors) have far less experience doing them. The end result: possibly lifesaving procedures are avoided in young children. Surprisingly, about three quarters of the states in this country do *not* require EMS workers to get continuing education in pediatric illness, according to a survey study published in the *Annals of Emergency Medicine*.[6]

Most emergency physicians and nurses have little or no formalized training in caring for seriously ill children. Incredibly, it is not rare for a hospital emergency department to lack proper equipment in sizes small enough for babies and young children. This is problematic since children are not miniature adults. They require precisely fitting masks, needles, tubes and other equipment.

Hospital emergency departments hire physicians, but rarely provide for them organized and formal reviews of what equipment is available, where equipment is stored and proper use of pediatric equipment. Imagine an emergency physician asking, "Where are the breathing tubes?" or "What tubes do we have?" when a child is blue and breathless on a stretcher.

Why is expert training in pediatric care needed? Serious illness in this age group differs from that in adults. Babies respond to illness in different ways. Children are at greater risk for serious breathing trouble and head injuries. A baby's body has little tolerance for blood loss, diarrhea or vomiting before going into shock. What's more, common clues to shock are often lacking in babies so doctors unfamiliar with baby care can and do underestimate serious illness in children. In an adult who is going into shock, the heart rate speeds up to over one hundred beats per minute and blood pressure falls below ninety. An infant's heart rate is already high and varies a great deal in the normal range. Furthermore, a baby's blood pressure often drops only in the final stages of shock, when death is imminent. Experience and special training are clearly needed when treating sick babies and young children.

PEDIATRIC NEAR MISSES IN THE ER

An example of the type of problems possible when bringing small children to the ER is evident in the following story.

A worried mother approached the emergency room registration desk toting her toddler on her hip. The boy's arms clung to his mother's torso like ivy to an old building.

"Can I help you?" the clerk asked.

"My baby was up all night coughing and isn't breathing right," the mother responded.

The desk clerk looked at the baby who rested his head on mother's shoulder, releasing his hug only to exhale a deep cough.

"How long has he been coughing?" the clerk asked.

"Since last night."

"Any fever?"

"No."

"Does the child have asthma?"

"No, but his older sister does."

"Have a seat, fill out these insurance forms then come back to the window."

The mother found a seat in the waiting area and the desk clerk printed out a chart listing the chief complaint as "cough." She handed the chart to the triage nurse who filed the minor complaint under the stack of patients-to-be-triaged charts.

Time passed slowly in the waiting room. The little boy began to grunt as his breathing became labored. The mother returned to the registration window and asked that her child be seen immediately. A few minutes later, the triage nurse (who sorts emergencies by how serious the illness is) called mother and child into the triage room. Removing only the baby's jacket, the nurse rested her pink stethoscope on the child's back—no audible wheezing. Temperature was normal. Pulse rate: 140—fast for a toddler. Respiratory rate: About forty-five, but difficult to measure between coughing spells. Any emergency room worker knows a baby's breathing rate is normally faster than an adult's average of fourteen breaths per minute. A child's breathing and heart rate are also likely to speed up at the sight of a white uniform. Preliminary impression: Bronchitis. Disposition: Sit out in the waiting room until called in order of arrival.

One by one patients were called through the metal emergency room doors. The mother nodded off with the baby on her lap. Suddenly her head snapped back and she let out a piercing scream, "My baby's turning blue! He's not breathing!" A doctor and nurse ran into the waiting area and saw the baby hanging limply in his mother's arms, his face grayish-blue, arms dangling, chest stationary. They raced him through the metal doors and placed an oxygen mask over the toddler's face, forcing air into his lungs. His skin color changed from gray to pink as oxygen-starved cells soaked up nutrients. The doctor listened with a stethoscope to the boy's chest and heard a cacophony of high-pitched wheezes. It was clear the boy was having a severe asthma attack.

Children often have just a cough as a sign of an asthma attack. Sometimes the attack is so severe the patient cannot breathe deeply enough to produce wheezes in the lungs, like blowing feebly into a trumpet with no sound emanating from the instrument. Had the triage nurse removed the boy's shirt and looked at his abnormal chest movements, with the muscles between ribs vigorously contracting, she would have recognized the breathing difficulty. Had the triage staff heeded the mother's concerns and done a more thorough examination of the boy, this near-calamity might have been prevented.

SIDESTEPPING THE PERILS FOR CHILDREN

One wrong decision by a parent or an emergency care professional can have irreversible consequences when serious illness or injury strikes a child. What can be done to minimize chances for sub-par care and maximize chances for quality medical care?

Basic Guidelines:

- Plan which nearby teaching hospital you will use in the event of medical calamity. Studies have confirmed that children who stop breathing or have serious head injuries have lower death rates if treated in hospitals having specialized pediatric intensive care. Those hospitals must have pediatric training programs and offer pediatric and neonatal intensive care units. Emergency departments ideally should have separate pediatric sections that are staffed by pediatricians. Only major teaching hospitals in big cities offer this. Those who live in areas remote from teaching hospitals have no choice but to go to the nearest hospital unless helicopter transport is available for serious injury or illness. Find out the location of the nearest hospital that offers helicopter transport for critical illness and injury.
- Use a pediatrician who is affiliated with a teaching hospital. Community hospitals tend to be less prepared and less experienced in treating seriously ill children. Teaching hospitals offer pediatric specialists in every field to advise or consult with your primary care pediatrician. Those who live in rural areas might not be able to see a pediatrician. Instead, a doctor trained in Family Medicine might be caring for these children. Bear in mind that Family Medicine doctors are jacks-of-all-trades and are not experts in treating babies and kids.
- Discuss with your pediatrician a plan of action for emergencies. What number should you call? What will be their availability? Where should you bring your child? How can you reach them after office hours?
- Keep a list of emergency telephone numbers handy, preferably near the telephone. You do not want to fumble around searching for a number while your child is very sick. Important numbers include ambulance (volunteer, paramedic or fire department), pediatricians, nearby hospital emergency rooms, local Poison Control Center, local police and neighbors to baby-sit your other children if you must seek help for one child. Find out if your community or one nearby has a paramedic unit available (perhaps through the fire department). They are the most skilled emergency field workers and are trained to perform many lifesaving procedures.
- Take a Basic Life Support (BLS) course that teaches proper handling of sick babies and children. This simple course can give you the

confidence to act with common sense and speed during a crisis and to differentiate between a true emergency and a scare. The American Heart Association or Red Cross Web sites offer BLS course information in your area. If you live in a remote location, consider purchasing a pediatric resuscitation kit that contains key life support equipment in child and baby sizes. Health professionals can then use your equipment if needed. Full resuscitation kits can be expensive so an alternative is to purchase a few individual masks and tubes (at your doctor's recommendation) from any medical supply catalog or Web site (Do a search using "medical supplies").

- If your child goes to a community hospital, it is important to get a pediatrician to come into the emergency room to care for your sick child. It can take several hours until a sick child is admitted and sent to a hospital bed or transferred to a university hospital for intensive care. You do not want your sick child to remain in the chaotic emergency department with little supervision, because a sick child's condition can quickly deteriorate. If your pediatrician or the on-call pediatrician won't come in to see your child, ask emergency staff to call another pediatrician.

- Do not make the common mistake of assuming that freestanding urgent care facilities have full emergency care capabilities. Many do not and these facilities are often not well prepared to treat serious or critical illness, particularly in babies or young children. For a very sick child (as opposed to a child with just a fever, earache, etc.) your best bet is to call your pediatrician first. If the illness is potentially life threatening, call an ambulance if one can respond within minutes. Do not drive your critically ill child to a hospital unless you live less than five minutes from a university emergency room.

Prevention of injuries and accidents is the most effective way to sidestep an emergency care system that inadequately cares for children. You cannot choose the competence of the ambulance technician, nurse or doctor who cares for your child. But you can work hard to minimize chances your child will be hurled into the unpredictable emergency care system. To a large extent, prevention *is* in your hands.

ANTICIPATE CHILDHOOD DANGERS
BEFORE THEY OCCUR

Balloons. Marbles. Coins. Vitamin supplements. Peanuts. These items hardly conjure up images of danger. But in the wrong hands—or mouths—they can be deadly. Children below age five eagerly explore their environment using the five senses. Their oral curiosity, however, puts them at risk, because they will put any object into their mouth. At times they may suck on an object because it resembles food or candy; sometimes they do it to explore or investigate; at other times they do it to mimic.

Choking as well as injuries, accidents, burns, drowning and poisonings account for a large proportion of death and disability among children. Parents must prevent these tragedies waiting to happen with proper information and hard work.

Choking

Buttons, hard candies and popcorn quickly lose their innocence when a child's face turns purplish-blue right in front of you. Toddlers are at greater risk for choking on foods because their back teeth (molars) have not yet erupted. Without these important teeth toddlers can have difficulty properly chewing foods such as hot dogs, grapes, carrots, nuts and certain beans. Hot dogs, nuts, seeds, and pieces of vegetable or fruit are the most common food causes for choking.

Foods are not the only choking hazards. The 1979 Consumer Products Safety Act banned toys with small parts for use in children under age three. Circular objects and small toys less than about 1.5 to 1.75 inches in diameter are not permitted in toys for kids below age three. But many common household objects can be hazardous to young children. Screws and bolts, pins, paper clips, rubber bands and coins cause many choking deaths and injuries as well. Round or cylinder-shaped objects such as marbles, hard candies and small balls are all high risk. Another culprit is the "button battery" found in electronics, cameras and watches. These small, round batteries can get lodged in the food tube or intestine and become toxic. Balloons were found in studies to be the most common cause of choking death in all children. Alarmingly, balloons can pose a greater risk for choking death in children older than three years of age!

When you purchase a toy for an older child, consider that your younger child will probably be around those small objects at an unsupervised moment. The lesson to be learned: You cannot watch an active toddler every moment of every day. Walk through your house and get rid of all small objects. Keep all coins, pills and hardware nuts and bolts in a locked cabinet. Never underestimate how nimbly kids can climb.

One important yet often overlooked method for prevention is as basic as parenting itself. Explain to children, even young toddlers, why they should not place small objects in their mouth. Telling children, "You might choke and get a bad boo-boo" might be an effective prevention technique for some kids, particularly with repetition. Studies have shown that even young children have some rudimentary understanding of abstract thinking and cause and effect. If nothing else, they might simply follow your rule.

Poisoning

Think of poisons and what comes to mind? Perhaps a skull and crossbones? Think again. There are many pretty poisons[7] sitting atop shelves, counters or tabletops. They are drugs or cleaning products to you, candy to curious Junior. Even poisons that do not look or smell appealing might be worth a taste for many toddlers.

You walk from room to room and remove toxic household products like Pine Sol, Drano, bleach and nail polish remover from the cabinets. You throw out or secure unused portions of motor oil, paint thinner, charcoal lighter fluid, turpentine, wood polish and antifreeze that are in the basement or garage. You remove all prescription pills from accessible night tables and purses. But it's just not enough. There are many "pretty" and plain poisons you might not consider to be hazardous.

Several iron supplements and multivitamins resemble M & M candies. Prenatal vitamins can resemble Good and Plenty candy. Aspergum resembles Chiclets gum. The amount of aspirin in Aspergum can cause harm to a child. Mothballs look similar to gumballs. Some dangerous alcohol-containing mouthwashes look like flavors of Kool-Aid. Pretty smells can also attract a child's culinary curiosity. Many toxic products smell like lemon, pine, Oil of Wintergreen or strawberry. Any product that can be dangerous to a child should be locked out of reach.

When you've locked away the obvious poisons do not overlook other ingestible hazards. Some of the most dangerous items sit atop tables and counters, remaining easy to reach for toddlers. Acetaminophen (Tylenol), aspirin, cold remedies, vitamin and iron supplements and alcohol can be deadly if enough is ingested.

Several common ingestions are surprising. Cosmetics, personal care products and plants are in the top five categories for poisoning exposures in young children. Fortunately, these ingestions are usually nontoxic or minimally toxic. Easy access, visually appealing packaging or lack of safety features can contribute to children's exposure to these products.

Simple Rules To Help Save Children's Lives

• Don't leave a drug out and lose a child. It only takes a minute while you are answering the phone or a doorbell ring for a child to swallow a dangerous substance.

• Parents must childproof any house they visit and remind their own visitors of good safety practices: all it takes is a five-minute discussion. Remember, about one-quarter of oral prescription drugs ingested by young kids belong to a person *not* living in their household! Visitors such as grandparents often bring medications with them in their purses or coat pockets. Grandparents, relatives and friends might leave these medications on countertops, night tables or in accessible drawers when children are visiting.

• Avoid taking medication in front of children. At the least, explain what you are doing and how they can get a "boo-boo" if they take your medicine, because it is *not* candy. Children imitate. If you pull off a cap with your teeth and mouth, they may do the same and more. If you take two blue pills and two white pills each morning, your child might want to also.

• Put over-the-counter (non-prescription) items like vitamins, aspirin, acetaminophen and cold remedies out of reach. These can be deadly to a child!

• Do not leave iron pills, which can be fatal to a child, where a child can get it. Iron is responsible for one-third of medication related poisoning deaths in kids, according to the Consumer Protection Services Commission. Iron can be found in the form of ferrous sulfate, ferrous gluconate, ferrous fumarate and in multivitamins with iron.

• Lock toxic items up. Do not rely on unlocked cabinets or drawers that seem to be out of reach. Kids climb and are quite resourceful.

• Do not depend on a child safety cap to stop your child from taking a prescription drug. The child might open the medication, even if the cap isn't already loose.

• Never switch storage containers. Do not put a toxic cleaner into an empty juice bottle, for instance.

• Administer Syrup of Ipecac, if indicated, to induce vomiting. This can be helpful in some poisonings if given within *one hour*. If a child ingests a handful of aspirin or iron pills, for instance, inducing vomiting promptly at home might be lifesaving. Some emergency and toxicology experts have questioned the effectiveness of Ipecac for poisoning. In fact, if used in the wrong type of poisoning Ipecac can be harmful. Keep a bottle in the house, out of reach of children, just in case your local Poison Control Center suggests using it. Poison Control can advise parents on whether or not to use Ipecac to induce vomiting, for example. General guidelines *not* to use Ipecac include a child who is drowsy or groggy, a child who is already vomiting and if the ingested substance is caustic like acid or lye.

• Bring all suspicious bottles with you to the emergency room so doctors know what was ingested.

If your child does ingest something while you are distracted and then you notice the child is having a medical problem, first check the child to be sure he or she is alert and breathing. If there is any indication of breathing difficulty or real drowsiness then call paramedics immediately to get your child to an emergency room. If the child vomits, scoop up any suspicious poisons or pill bottles and seek care at an emergency room. If the child seems unharmed, look around for open bottles or loose pills. Ask the child what she ate and how many. If it is not clear that the child did ingest something (he or she might deny it, fearing punishment), check for clues of a poison ingestion. Look for residue in the teeth and mouth or on the lips. Check for burns. Smelling the child's breath can provide clues as well.

Not all ingestions are toxic so the majority of poisonings can be safely handled at home. If the child seems unharmed gather suspicious bottles and call the Poison Control Center. The number should already be posted near your telephone. If it is not handy, you can find the number on the inside cover of the Yellow or White Pages or get it from the American Association of Poison Control Centers Web site.

Many doctors and nurses, in fact, consult with Poison Control for advice and information. Poison Control has the latest information available on what ingredients are found in household products and the most effective treatments.

Appendicitis In Children

Appendicitis is easily missed in young children. Like in older adults, appendicitis in children is difficult to diagnose because symptoms are usually less typical, the patient often cannot provide an accurate account of symptoms, other illness complaints can confuse the diagnosis and perforation rates are high, especially in children under two years of age.

Initial symptoms of appendicitis in young children are fussiness, irritability, loss of interest in playing, crying, vomiting, abdominal bloating and abdominal pain in children old enough to verbalize it.

Those who can verbalize their symptoms will typically complain of pain around the belly button region that within hours moves to the lower right part of the abdomen. Additional facts you should know about appendicitis in children:

- This abdominal emergency is unusual in infants, but has a high death rate when it happens.
- In children under age two years, the death rate from appendicitis can be as high as fifty percent.
- The perforation rate in those under age two years approaches one hundred percent.
- A child suffering from an attack of appendicitis will not want to move or cough because it increases the abdominal pain.
- Gastroenteritis (food poisoning or stomach virus) is the most common misdiagnosis in children who have appendicitis. Beware of this diagnosis in a child who has vomiting only, diarrhea and vomiting and in those with small mucousy bowel movements. Gastroenteritis usually causes frequent *large volume* stools. Other family members or close contacts might have just had similar symptoms. A stomach virus is often accompanied by rash or higher fevers as well.
- In about half of the cases of misdiagnosed appendicitis, the patient will have complained of maximal tenderness in the lower right part of the abdomen. Do not let a doctor ignore or dismiss this finding on examination.
- Pain nearly always *precedes* nausea or vomiting with an attack of appendicitis. In children, however, this is less reliable. Children may not complain of pain when it first develops and vomiting may be the parent's first clue the child is truly ill.
- Upper respiratory cold symptoms such as head congestion, throat irritation, and cough are often present along with appendicitis in children. What's more, "Strep" throat can itself cause abdominal pain. Never allow your child's belly pain to be dismissed just because the child has some upper respiratory symptoms too. If that "cold" seems to have made your child much more ill than usual, be sure a doctor reevaluates the abdomen within several hours if the belly pain persists or your child appears worse.

GIVING MEDICATION TO CHILDREN

Whether prescribed by your family physician or an ER doctor or when you feel your child's mild illness will be helped by an over-the-counter product, giving medication to a child is more than science and more than art: it's a challenge. The catchphrase to keep in mind is *kids are not little adults*. Children can be divided into five age categories, each with its unique features based on how a child's body works at different stages of development. The five age categories are:

1. Newborn to thirty days old
2. One to twelve months old (infant)
3. One to four years old (toddler)
4. Five to twelve years old (child)
5. Above twelve years of age (adolescent)

Both the liver and kidneys process medications in the body. The concentration of a drug can depend on such factors as body weight, percent of muscle versus fat, availability of certain enzymes to break down drugs, amount of protein in the blood and other medications in the body. By age six months, an infant's kidneys work on par with that of an adult and by three years of age, a toddler's kidneys work even more efficiently. A one-year-old has better liver function than adults so certain medications would have to be given in *relatively* larger doses or more frequently than for an adult.

Another example of how a child's body changes over time is the amount of body fat. A newborn has about twelve percent body fat while a one-year-old has thirty percent body fat. An average adult body is made up of approximately eighteen percent body fat. The amount of body fat affects how a drug works in the body.

The person getting a medication must also have the necessary "machinery" to process the substance. Infants do not take well to codeine (a narcotic pain medicine and cough suppressant), because they do not have enough of the needed enzyme that processes that drug. Small amounts of codeine or even dextromethorphan (the DM in cough remedies) can cause an infant's breathing to stop. In another example of body differences, children under age three have less stomach acid than adults. That higher stomach pH will allow penicillin to be better absorbed while commonly used acetaminophen will *not* get absorbed as efficiently.

In a hospital or emergency room, be particularly vigilant when your child is given medication. Learn the medication names, doses and reasons they are needed. Weigh your child since they grow quickly and dosages are determined by the child's size. Watch out for the all too common but dangerous "decimal point" error in calculating pediatric doses which are based on a child's weight. This error occurs when, for example, 2.0 milligrams of a drug are given instead of 0.2 milligrams. That is a dosage ten times higher than what is called for.

Even topical creams and ointments can have significant effects on young children. A child's skin is thinner and more sensitive than that of an adult so more topical medication penetrates through the skin's protective barrier. Open skin is particularly susceptible to a drug entering the body in higher than expected concentration. An area of irritation or eczema or a wound will allow greater drug penetration into a child's body. What's more, covering an area of skin where medication was applied, a technique doctors call occlusion, can greatly increase the amount of drug that enters the body. A diaper can create a similar occlusive effect so be careful of medications and their amounts that you rub on baby's bottom. Besides, babies might wipe some medication off and lick it off their hands, which increase the amount of the drug in baby's system. A child also has a greater surface area of skin relative to their weight so topical drugs can have a greater effect on young children.

Five Key Aspects to Successfully Medicating a Child
- Ask yourself, "Is a medication truly necessary?"
- Use the correct medication
- Measure doses accurately
- Use age appropriate technique to give medication
- Use ways to enhance its taste

Minimizing Side Effects
Young children are especially susceptible to side effects from medication. A baby's cold symptoms would likely benefit more from suctioning baby's nose than from an over-the-counter cold remedy, for instance. That same medication could transform a slightly grouchy baby into a highly irritable one. Be selective about giving young children medication of any kind including over-the-counter and herbal remedies.

Avoiding Drug Risks
Avoid codeine and dextromethorphan (DM) in infants, for instance, unless your doctor specifically instructs you to use it in small doses. The risks of these drugs are too high for casual use in infants. Do not use multi-ingredient remedies when all you really need is acetaminophen to reduce fever. Do not use aspirin to reduce fever in children because of the risk for Reye's syndrome, a rare but fatal complication of aspirin use during certain viral illnesses. Avoid using decongestants in infants since they can cause irritability. If decongestants (chemically related to

'speed' or amphetamines) can cause insomnia, restlessness or palpitations in adults, just imagine the possible effects of this drug on infants.

Placing medication into a bottle other than the original container is a common cause for mistakenly giving the wrong medication. Don't switch bottles.

Giving Children Proper Dosages

You might be setting yourself up for disaster if you give your child smaller amounts of adult remedies. Even if you do not make errors, your mother-in-law, spouse, or baby-sitter might one day inadvertently overdose your child. Use over-the-counter remedies formulated specifically for children.

One reminder worth writing down before you go to the pediatrician's office is to ask for a three ml or five ml graded syringe (without the needle). You should keep a couple handy even if your child does not need medication that particular visit. Immediately after opening the syringe, toss out the small syringe cap since it is a choking hazard. Avoid using a kitchen teaspoon for giving medication since there is significant variation in the actual amount of liquid in each kitchen teaspoon. In general, one teaspoon is equal to five milliliters (or cc's) while one tablespoon equals fifteen milliliters (or three teaspoons).

Use a real medical syringe not measuring cups and bulb syringes which may be lying around the house. Most pediatric medications have a thick, gooey (viscous) consistency. If you place the suspension into a cup or bulb syringe, a large portion of it will stick to the sides or bottom. A significant percentage of the dose will be lost. The same holds true for putting bitter-tasting medication into a bottle, cup or portion of food. If junior does not want to finish his portion, the medication is lost. What's more, lots of medication is lost when the child spits up part of the dose. Using a syringe with proper technique is more likely to get the full dose into baby.

Helping the Child Take Medications

Babies and young toddlers typically give the most resistance to taking their medication. The solution is not as simple as "a spoon full of sugar," but this advice can help. Many common medications are available in liquid or suspension form and have flavors added to improve taste. If you know your child despises one particular medication and routinely spits it out that would be your first step toward the solution. Ask the doctor if there is an alternative medication that is effective.

If your child routinely spits out absolutely any medication, your next approach is to use ER nurse technique for a baby or sweet ingenuity for a toddler. The technique is simple: Prepare the dosage of medication in a syringe. Put the baby on a bed lying flat. If he or she is a screamer and fighter, have someone stand at baby's head holding hands and arms up alongside the cheeks to limit head movements. The one giving the medication should gently squeeze the baby's cheeks to pry open the mouth and squirt about one cc into the cheek of one side, then gently push baby's chin up to close the mouth and prevent spitting up the medication. When that dose is swallowed squirt another one cc of medication into the other cheek—not the back of baby's throat because the gag reflex will cough it all up—and press the chin up to close baby's mouth. Repeat until all medication is swallowed. Another tip to make this procedure simpler is to ask your doctor to prescribe a more concentrated dose, if available, so you need give only half the amount of liquid to baby.

For toddlers who get tossed into a tizzy when medication is on the menu, there are several tricks of the trade you can try. Chill the liquid or suspension if refrigeration is allowed. It might help prevent spoilage of the medication and bitter-tasting medication is easier to swallow when cold. Chilling liquid medication might also lessen a medication's bad odor.

If the chilled medication trick is not enough, try sweetening the taste by adding chocolate syrup, fruit punch or applesauce. Ask your pharmacist if any of these tasty additives will affect the active ingredient.

Additional Tips for Administering Medication to Children

- Kids often do not like chewable medication because the taste lingers longer. Also, be alert for choking when a child uses chewable medication.
- If you must crush a pill and put it in applesauce or other more palatable food, ask your doctor or pharmacist if that is permitted since coated and extended release formulations should not be crushed.
- Milk can cause coated medication to dissolve in the stomach, not the intestine where it should dissolve. Wash down coated pills with an acidic juice like apple or cranberry. Purified or distilled water, of course, is safest when in doubt.
- Beware of alcohol in many over-the-counter remedies and mouthwashes. That alcohol can be toxic to young children who drink it.

- Ask your doctor to write about thirty cc's of extra medication on the prescription to account for medication spillage and spit-up. You would be surprised how many doctors write for exactly the amount of medication needed.
- If your baby has a bad reaction to a medication, he or she might show it only with irritability, being fussy, vomiting, some other change in behavior or not eating.
- Know your child's recent weight.
- One teaspoon = five ml; 1 tablespoon = fifteen ml
- Children can take 100-150 milligrams of acetaminophen (Tylenol) for each twenty-two pounds of weight (acetaminophen: every four to six hours, no more than five doses per twenty-four hours). Ibuprofen can be given in doses of ten to twenty milligrams for each pound of weight (every six to eight hours, no more than four maximal doses per twenty-four hours). During active illness, it is better to give the medication around the clock to minimize wide temperature swings. Measure pediatric doses carefully using graded droppers, measuring utensils or, better still, a syringe.
- Avoid giving aspirin to children with a fever who are under age sixteen years unless your doctor specifically advises you to use aspirin. Aspirin use in kids suffering from a flu-like illness or chicken pox has been associated with brain and liver damage—the deadly Reye's syndrome. Acetaminophen and ibuprofen are safer and equally effective alternatives.
- Most importantly, do not leave these remedies within reach of children! Acetaminophen and aspirin can be deadly if taken in high dosages (ten or more times the usual dose).
- Before using over-the-counter cold remedies in young children and babies, try giving the child a warm bath or nasal suction. If you use a humidifier, clean it frequently (daily or every other day) so bacteria do not collect in the well.
- For better vision when measuring doses—keep a magnifying glass handy.
- Check for any sign of tampering on over-the-counter medications such as punctures or an open safety seal.
- Always look inside and check for signs of degradation or spoilage such as discolored pills or liquid and strange consistency or odor.

To expand your abilities to avoid pediatric perils and to handle those that do happen with strength and knowledge, make use of the following Web sites.

USEFUL WEB SITES

Child Safety
http://www.imsafe.com
   (The I'm Safe Network helps parents and educators keep children safe from the leading cause of death: unintentional injuries.)

http://www.kidsafe.org
   (Homepage of the National Safe Kids Campaign, an effort to reduce unintentional injuries and make the world safer for children.)

http://www.nhtsa.dot.gov/people/injury/childps
   (Information on proper car safety seat usage for children of varying ages and weights.)

http://www.nlm.nih.gov/medlineplus/childsafety.html
   (Articles containing the latest news, topical information, prevention and research in child safety.)

http://www.cpsc.gov/cpscpub/pubs/chld_sfy.html
   (Documents on product alerts as well as child safety tips and guidelines for parents from the Consumer Product Safety Commission.)

CPR, Choking and First Aid
http://www.learn-cpr.com
http://www.learncpr.org
   (Both Web sites have information and instructions on performing first aid for choking victims and CPR on adults, children and infants.)

http://www.cprplusnet.com
   (Provides a listing of CPR classes by state.)

http://www.cpr-ecc.org
   (Information on CPR from the American Heart Association.)

http://www.healthcentral.com/mhc/top/000011.cfm
   (Information and how to do CPR on infants.)

http://www.healthcentral.com/mhc/top/000012.cfm
   (Information and how to do CPR on kids age one to eight years.)

http://www.healthcentral.com/mhc/top/000013.cfm
   (Information and how to do CPR on kids older than eight years.)

http://www.redcross.org
(Web site lists First Aid and CPR courses offered by the Red Cross.)

http://www.aapcc.org
(American Association of Poison Control Centers' Web site.)

Medical Supplies:
http://www.hmponline.com

http://www.allmed.net/catalog

http://www.medcom1.com

5

EMERGENCY ROOM ALTERNATIVES: WHERE ELSE CAN I TURN?

A teenager cuts his hand the first time he uses a power tool. The cut doesn't look too deep. Should mom rush him to an emergency room? Are there other options? A man experiences a mild asthma attack. Where can he go for help to avoid emergency room havoc? Two months after a woman undergoes heart surgery, she experiences chest pains and difficulty breathing. Where should she go for medical care?

There was a time when people could count on their family doctors to make house calls if they became ill. A generation ago, a family doctor might have driven a patient to the hospital if the illness seemed serious. Medical care has changed. As family doctors became less available to patients and more people became uninsured, patient visits to emergency rooms skyrocketed. Overcrowding at emergency rooms has sent waiting times into orbit and quality of care has suffered as a result.

Primary care doctors began to provide out-of-hospital care that was a cross between a doctor's office and small emergency room. These offices were called "urgent care" or "immediate care" centers. Open up to fifteen hours each day, six or seven days a week, they have become a great convenience for patients who need sudden, immediate care for mild to moderate illnesses.

Today, many family practice physicians provide both urgent and ongoing care. Doctors trained in Family Practice (and Emergency Medicine) are true primary care doctors. They do minor surgery, gynecological care, treat babies and children and handle ailments ranging from sore throats to heart attacks.

Primary care doctors who are trained in Internal Medicine, Family Practice or Emergency Medicine typically staff urgent care offices. These primary care doctors can provide limited and basic care in a variety of specialties. The sickest patients must be transported from the office to a hospital. Many patients are also referred to specialists for complex surgical, eye, heart or other specialty care.

Where should the teen who cut his hand be treated? Since it happened during office hours, it might be possible for his family doctor to evaluate the cut and send him directly to a specialist, if needed. The man who suffers from mild asthma attacks enjoys quick and adequate treatment at his community urgent care center. He used to spend hours at the emergency room, needlessly getting poked with needles. On the other hand, the woman with a history of heart disease who experienced chest pains should go to an emergency room, preferably at the hospital where the surgery was performed and where her cardiologist has admitting privileges. Since she carries in her pocketbook a miniaturized, laminated copy of her baseline electrocardiogram, however, even if she is taken to an unfamiliar hospital, the doctors there can compare her old to a new electrocardiogram to detect subtle changes.

The lesson to be learned: Get the right person for the right job. If an illness is possibly serious and you have chronic medical problems like diabetes, high blood pressure or heart disease, seek help at an emergency room. You will probably be sent there anyway. For less serious illness or injury or for problems present for several days or more, four good alternatives to emergency rooms exist:

- Urgent or immediate care center
- Family practice office
- Specialist's office
- Private doctor's office

URGENT CARE FACILITY/FAMILY PRACTICE OFFICE

An urgent care facility or family practice office can provide fine care or inept care. Each office is only as good as the physicians and nurses who work there. Treatment at an urgent care office is typically focused on one new problem that led you to seek medical assistance. A family practice office might also provide ongoing patient care and manage chronic illnesses such as diabetes or high blood pressure.

How can you know if a particular office is ethical and provides quality care? Follow recommendations from reliable friends, relatives or neighbors in your community. Physicians at these practices should be evaluated in the same way you would evaluate an emergency room doctor. Board certification in a specialty is one *unreliable* measure of quality since all it means is that doctor studied notes and passed a written test. Hospital affiliations by an urgent care center might be helpful, but it might mean that only one doctor in the practice holds admitting privileges at the affiliated hospital. It is still no guarantee that the doctor who treats you is skilled and experienced. Do not base your decision solely on isolated Better Business Bureau complaints or malpractice suits since nobody can please *all* patients *all* of the time. A *long* list of complaints or lawsuits, however, is likely to be useful information.

Another measure of a quality urgent care office is staffing by registered nurses, board-certified physicians and licensed X-ray technicians. Adequate follow-up care is also important in a quality practice. Follow-up care includes phone calls to check on your condition and to report test results. Necessary return visits are important to check for progress or to detect deterioration, particularly for such problems as abdominal pain, lacerations or bad infections. A quality practice should also provide ready access to specialist care when appropriate.

If you choose an office based on these criteria and your experience proves satisfying, that is wonderful. There are dangers, however, as well as advantages to seeking medical care at urgent care facilities.

Reasons to Seek Out Alternative Facilities

- Urgent Care offices are open ten to fifteen hours, six or seven days each week, including most holidays. This is a priceless convenience when your private doctor cannot fit you into the schedule or is out of town.
- These practices often treat patients who have minor fractures, sprains and cuts that do not need specialist care, but that general internists and pediatricians do *not* treat.
- Waiting time until you receive care will be far shorter than at most emergency rooms.
- Fees are generally much lower than costs for emergency room care.
- Patient satisfaction is important to urgent medical care providers since they prosper when people come back. Emergency room workers, on the other hand, might feel there are far too many patients.
- If you are satisfied with one particular doctor's style of care at an urgent care practice, you can go there when that doctor is on duty.

Reasons to Avoid Alternative Facilities

- The most serious danger that an urgent care facility or a family practice office poses is that it can be a cause for treatment delay. Patients often mistakenly seek care at these offices for serious problems such as heart attack or stroke, trying to "avoid the hospital." Learning both the common and less typical symptoms of stroke and heart attack can help people avoid this error.
- Another serious error is the misconception that these offices or facilities are well-equipped enough to treat seriously ill babies and young children. Big Mistake! Most nurses and doctors who staff these facilities have minimal, if any, training or experience treating seriously ill children. Many offices even lack critical care equipment!
- Urgent care or family practice offices prosper from high patient volume. A busy office can have nearly one hundred people hobbling through each day. That translates into fleeting doctor-patient encounters. It can be frustrating when a doctor interrupts the one or two sentences you manage to utter to hurry you along.
- There is generally high doctor turnover at these practices. What's more, each doctor's training and skill varies greatly, sometimes resulting in an inconsistent quality of care.
- Payment is expected at the time care is rendered; emergency rooms will bill you. Check if the urgent care practice you want to use accepts your health insurance. Even if you must pay cash up front, care is far less expensive than it would cost at an emergency room.
- As a general rule, be wary of the fee-for-service setup in which each test ordered or procedure performed brings an additional charge. Whether at an emergency room, urgent care facility, or doctor's office, the more tests or procedures performed the more money generated. Doctors surely have added incentive to do more whether the tests are truly necessary or not. Remember this simple equation: more tests + more procedures = more income + greater patient risk.
- Healthy skepticism is useful when a doctor wants to do a test, X ray or procedure. Use the same emergency room guidelines to screen unnecessary tests in an urgent care facility. *Will the test change the treatment plan? What risks and alternatives exist? Would it be prudent to simply watch and wait?*
- Be suspicious of an urgent care facility or family practice office that does not refer you to a specialist for more complex lacerations, fractures

or other medical illness. An inexperienced doctor might treat your complex laceration, for instance, without proper expertise.

- A corollary to the above guideline is to proceed with caution when an urgent care or family practice office refers you for specialized testing that is done by that *same* office. Stress tests, echocardiograms, sigmoidoscopy screening, sonograms and other special tests can be a great source of income for a practice. But you must carefully evaluate if the test is truly needed. Would the doctor order the test if you were going to have it done at an outside radiology or specialist office? More importantly, tests are only as good as the people who perform and interpret them. For instance, have your stress test done at a skilled cardiologist's office. This doctor has expertise interpreting the results and following up with your care.

- Some doctors at urgent care practices prescribe needless antibiotics and other treatments to make patients "happy" to get treatment. These so-called "happy" patients come back—usually with more side effects than satisfaction. Do not fall into the "We must treat everything" trap. Any treatment can have serious side effects.

SPECIALIST'S OFFICE

Direct care from quality specialists can be very valuable. They are experts in treating your particular type of illness or injury. Go directly to an orthopedist for a bad bone or joint injury, especially if you are an athlete. A pianist needs the expertise of a hand surgeon even for a moderate hand injury. If you cut your hand during the daytime while using a power tool, going directly to a hand surgeon might be prudent. A woman with a previous heart attack should call her cardiologist for any chest pains or unusual indigestion. When an active toddler sustains a gash across his forehead, a trip straight to a plastic surgeon would be a wise decision.

There are, however, a few concerns. Specialists are hard to reach, particularly during the night or on weekends. They often do surgery or procedures during the day, making them unavailable for many hours. Going to a specialist sometimes results in having a procedure performed whether absolutely necessary or not, simply because that is what they do. In addition, specialist care does not come cheaply. Each visit or procedure may cost hundreds to thousands of dollars so be sure to see a quality specialist who participates in your health plan. Many insurance policies require that you get a referral from your primary care doctor before seeing a specialist. This can, at times, be frustrating and cause delays. Read your insurance manual to find out your policy's rules and restrictions.

PRIVATE DOCTOR'S OFFICE

When you fall ill your family doctor can be your most important ally. Will your family doctor promptly return your phone call for urgent advice? Or squeeze you into a busy office schedule? Will he or she get out of bed at 2:00 A.M. to care for you in the emergency room? Do not count on it if you have not established a tight doctor-patient bond.

Know your family doctor well and he or she will feel obliged to take the extra step for you. Go for annual checkups and screening examinations. Share some of your personal life with your doctor. A devoted family doctor is invaluable.

ADVANTAGES OF A STRONG DOCTOR-PATIENT BOND

- Your appropriate phone calls will be answered within a reasonable amount of time.
- Your doctor can advise you on using simple home remedies and symptoms for which to look out. He or she can provide specialist referrals when needed. Letting your doctor know you sustained a gash across your forehead, for instance, might produce a quick and direct referral to see a plastic surgeon during daytime hours.
- If an urgent office visit is warranted, your family doctor will often squeeze you into a busy schedule.
- If an illness requires hospital evaluation, your doctor might meet you at the emergency room or, if needed, directly admit you into the hospital.
- Your family doctor will be familiar with your baseline health, personal habits, preferences and reliability in complying with treatment. He or she will be more willing to work with you to avoid hospital admission using close outpatient follow up care.
- A quality family doctor will keep records of all screening and preventive care you have gotten at different stages of life.

Though family doctors are advisable, there are several good options available for getting quality urgent medical care. Consider these options for less serious illnesses and injuries, before you rush through those large, metal emergency room doors. One never knows what will happen inside.

CONCLUSION

Although the intention of all emergency medical care systems is to provide excellent treatment to all who enter their doors, too often that goal is not reached. While most ER staffs are comprised of dedicated professionals, overwork and high levels of stress frequently contribute to poor patient care, poor diagnosis and, perhaps, rushed judgements in the ER setting.

Receiving high quality care in an emergency medical facility depends to a great degree on you, whether you are a patient, a parent or serve as a healthcare advocate for a loved one. The very nature of an emergency illness or injury means it is unanticipated; however, you have the ability to lay the groundwork upon which solid emergency care can be built. What determines success or failure is your level of preparedness.

Research the emergency care facilities in your area. Compile a list of recommended physician specialists. Establish a good relationship with your family or primary care doctor. Learn the pros and cons of commonly utilized tests and procedures. Doing these things will make you an educated emergency medical care consumer. Questioning the ER physician about your diagnosis and proposed tests or procedures and remembering you have the option to refuse or postpone a suggested plan of action will allow you input and management of your own healthcare.

Reading *ER: Enter at Your Own Risk* has acquainted you with the dangers that lurk inside our emergency rooms and advised you how to combat them. It has provided tips for knowing when you or a family member needs to seek emergency care and, once there, how to be a helpful ER advocate who contributes to the success of your or your loved one's medical care. The section on Pediatric Perils was designed to give parents the confidence to avoid panic and the knowledge to make sensible decisions when faced with their worst nightmare—a sick or injured child.

Keep this guide through the emergency medical care system handy and refer to it when needed. Despite hopes that sudden and severe illnesses or injuries will not strike you or family members, they can and will. Be prepared. Arm yourself with knowledge and mastery of the risks—before you enter the ER.

APPENDIX

A

COMMON EMERGENCY ROOM STAFF

Healthcare Provider is the person who is primarily responsible for overseeing your medical care. That person can be a Doctor (MD or DO), Nurse Practitioner, Physician Assistant, Doctor-in-training or Medical Student.

Triage Nurse is a specially trained RN who screens patients to decide upon their priority for evaluation. They weed out the routine medical care problems and less serious patients from true emergencies.

RN (Registered Nurse) is the person who will oversee your moment-to-moment care, dispense and administer medication, insert intravenous lines and be on the front line of patient monitoring and care.

Medical or Nurse's Assistant will assist nurses with basic duties such as patient hygiene and personal needs and performing electrocardiograms, drawing blood, stocking supplies and checking vital signs.

Desk Clerk is responsible for paperwork duties. The screening receptionist who takes insurance information might serve as the first person to "evaluate" people at some emergency rooms. They will call a nurse over if a person who is registering mentions an "alarm" symptom like chest pain.

Specialists are specially trained doctors who are called to the ER by emergency room healthcare providers to treat more complex illness and injury, to perform special procedures or to admit patients into the hospital. Specialists can be experienced or, at teaching hospitals, might be Fellows who are inexperienced and learning that specialty or Resident doctors-in-training.

B

SPECIALISTS

A specialist is a doctor who serves as a consultant to care for patients with more complex illnesses or injuries. These experts will be called upon by either an emergency room doctor, a patient's family doctor or the patient may request evaluation by a specialist. They are called for a second opinion, to admit patients into the hospital or to perform a procedure or surgery.

Anesthesiologists are experts in pain control during surgery and in managing breathing crises.

Cardiologists have expert training in treating heart ailments. Some cardiologists perform invasive surgical procedures like angioplasty, while others do more medically-oriented medical practice.

Dermatologists are uncommonly needed in the emergency room setting.

Ear, Nose and Throat doctors manage breathing crises and ailments involving the ears, nose and throat.

Gastroenterologists are the medical experts in treating diseases of the stomach, intestines, liver, gallbladder and pancreas—which together comprise the digestive tract or gastrointestinal system.

General Surgeons perform many bread and butter operations like appendectomy and hernia repair; they may also be trauma (injury) care experts.

Infectious Disease (ID) doctors know all about the many perplexing infections including HIV.

Internal Medicine doctors are specialists that have been branded as primary care doctors who treat anything from abdominal pain to zits. They are the "diagnosticians."

Neurologists know all the workings of the brain, spinal cord and nerves.

Neurosurgeons know what neurologists know and operate to repair injuries, remove tumors, clip aneurysms, etc.

Obstetricians/Gynecologists treat diseases of the female reproductive tract and deliver babies. They perform surgery when needed.

Ophthalmologists treat eye problems medically and surgically.

Pediatricians care for babies and children. **Neonatologists** are pediatricians with further expertise treating newborns and premature babies.

Plastic Surgeons are experts in wound care and aesthetics. They might treat severe burns, facial lacerations, disfiguring injuries, severe infections and perform elective cosmetic surgery.

Podiatrists medically and surgically care for foot disorders.

Psychiatrists treat serious mental illness in the emergency room including suicidal, psychotic and violent people.

Pulmonologists are experts at lung diseases and care of the critically ill.

Radiologists perform and interpret tests involving X-ray, CAT scan, MRI and Nuclear Medicine technology. Interventional radiologists perform surgical procedures involving X-ray technology and catheters (tubes inserted into the body).

Rheumatologists are experts in bone, joint and muscle diseases.

Trauma Surgeons have extra training in treating severe injuries such as gunshot wounds and the traumas sustained in serious motor vehicle accidents.

Urologists treat disorders of the male and female genital and urinary systems using medical and surgical approaches.

Vascular Surgeons surgically treat disorders of blood vessels.

APPENDIX
C

STOCKING YOUR MEDICINE CHEST WITH COMMONLY NEEDED REMEDIES

Americans are four times more likely to buy an over-the-counter remedy than to consult a doctor for an illness, according to the American Pharmaceutical Association. Over-the-counter remedies serve several key functions. They offer convenience by allowing the ill person to avoid a doctor's visit or to quickly get symptomatic relief while waiting for an appointment to see a doctor. These remedies also empower people by allowing for self-care, enabling individuals to take an active role in their own care.

Over-the-counter remedies are not without dangers. These remedies can mask symptoms of more serious underlying illness, thereby delaying proper treatment. Furthermore, these remedies can aggravate medical conditions such as high blood pressure, glaucoma or prostate problems. Some of these remedies can seriously impair driving or work performance and concentration. Bearing these risks in mind, health consumers must read labels carefully and respect dosage and length of use limits mentioned on the label. Most over-the-counter remedies advise discontinuation or seeing a doctor after three to ten days of use, depending on the particular remedy.

So how can a health consumer decide what remedies they should use? It is not as complicated as it may appear. What it comes down to is forgetting all the brand names that have been subliminally placed into your mind. While there exist hundreds of cold or pain remedies, there are only a handful of ingredients in them that perform the desired function. FDA approved generic versions of these remedies should work just as well as heavily advertised brands. Think function—what do I need that remedy to do for me? Once you have answered that question, you will be able to choose one of just a few different active ingredients for that purpose. This will save you money as well as allowing you to avoid medications with multiple active ingredients which you don't need and which could lead to unpleasant side effects.

Medicine Chest Necessities

You will want to have effective remedies readily available for commonly encountered ailments to avoid 3:00 A.M. trips to an emergency room or all-night pharmacy. Some of the most common active ingredients in over-the-counter or prescription medicines are:

1. **Pain or fever**
   - Aspirin
   - Acetaminophen
   - Ibuprofen
   - Naproxen
   - Ketoprofen
2. **Cough and cold symptoms**
   - Dextromethorphan (DM) – cough suppressant
   - Guaifenesin – mucous thinner
   - Acetaminophen – fever and pain reducer
   - Pseudoephedrine or Phenylephrine – decongestants
3. **Allergies and allergic reactions**
   - First generation antihistimines are over-the-counter and usually cause drowsiness: Chlorpheniramine, Brompheniramine, Tripolidine, Diphenhydramine, Carbinoxamine, Clemsatine, Azatadine, Cyproheptadine, Promethazine.
   - Second generation antihistamines do not cause drowsiness, but are currently only available by prescription (there has been a recent push to make them over-the-counter): Loratidine, Fexofenadine.
4. **Nausea/Vomiting Remedies**
   - Ingredients in prescription medicines are the most effective: Prochlorperazine, Trimethobenzamide, Hydroxyzine, Promethazine.
5. **Diarrhea Remedies**
   - Loperamide
   - Bismuth subsalicylate
   - Attapulgite
   - Electrolyte-rich sports drinks and salty crackers are good anti-dehydration and replacement foods.

Other common over-the-counter remedies that should be stocked in a medicine chest:

- Anti-fungal remedies for skin infections such as jock itch and athlete's foot, diaper rash, and vaginal yeast infections.
- Anti-itch topical remedies with hydrocortisone, a mild steroid and anti-inflammatory ingredient.
- Laxatives for significant constipation that is not caused by a treatable medical condition.
- Antacids and acid-lowering medication for heartburn or dyspepsia.
- Topical pain liquids to help such unexpected problems as dental pain until proper treatment can be sought.
- Antiseptics and anti-bacterials for minor cuts and scrapes.
- Consider keeping an adrenaline shot auto-injector handy for life-threatening allergic reactions. This is a vital part of the medicine chest when a family member has had a bad allergic reaction to food or insect venom.

Other items to include in the medicine chest are:
- Gauze and bandages
- Surgical tape
- Scissors
- Tweezers or hemostat (scissor with gripping teeth) to remove ticks and splinters
- Cotton balls

Another key concept to bear in mind while stocking your medicine chest is to include certain prescription drugs too. It is reasonable to keep a few codeine or hydrocodone pills handy for a pain crisis, particularly if you have a history of kidney stones, toothaches, or lower back problems, for example. You must exercise caution when asking your doctor for these medications so there is no misunderstanding that you are seeking narcotic drugs.

Few over-the-counter remedies are available for vomiting. Ask your doctor for a prescription anti-nausea remedy to keep handy.

Keeping certain prescription drugs handy for ailments to which you are susceptible might one day help to prevent an avoidable emergency room visit.

USEFUL WEB SITES:

http://www.panhealth.com

(PanHealth offers personalized services like healthcare planning, personal data management and scheduling of doctor appointments.)

http://www.e-eldercare.com

(E-Eldercare provides services to families caring for elderly parents or relatives such as locating housing, coordinating care needs, family counseling and financial monitoring.)

http://www.epill.com

(E-pill offers a wide range of medication management products, programs and services to help patients remember to take medications.)

http://www.medreminder.com

(Medreminder offers a paging service to help patients remember to take medications.)

http://www.ascp.com

(The American Society of Consultant Pharmacists is dedicated to advancing the practice of senior care pharmacy and improving the lives of geriatric patients.)

http://www.fda.gov

(The Food and Drug Administration's Web site provides various information including safety alerts and newly approved products.)

http://www.ismp.org

(The Institute for Safe Medication Practices researches and provides information on adverse drug events and their prevention in an effort to make these products safer for the public.)

http://dietary-supplements.info.nih.gov

(Under the National Institutes of Health, the Office of Dietary Supplements explores how supplements can improve healthcare. The Web site includes a database of over 400,000 dietary supplements.)

APPENDIX

D

ER VISIT LOG

Date Arrived _____ Date Left _____

Patient _____

Hospital _____

Ambulance Needed   Y _____ N _____

Treating Doctors and Titles _____

_____

_____

Nurses _____

_____

Specialists and Type of Specialty _____

_____

Diagnosis _____

_____

Admitted to Hospital   Y _____ N _____

Blood Tests and Results _____

_____

X rays and Results _____

_____

EKG and Results_____

_____

Other Diagnostic Tests and Results_____

_____

Major Procedures/Operations_____

_____

Minor Procedures _____

_____

Common Tests and Treatments

Heart Monitor	Y _____	N_____
EKG	Y _____	N_____
Oxygen	Y _____	N_____
Intravenous	Y _____	N_____
MRI/CT SCAN	Y _____	N_____
Pulse Oximeter (O_2 level)	Y _____	N_____
Urinary Catheter	Y _____	N_____
Nebulizer	Y _____	N_____

Medications Given (indicate oral or IV)_____

_____

Tests Refused_____

_____

Medications Refused _____

_____

Tests Repeated and Reasons Why _____

_____

Overall Evaluation of the ER Experience _____

_____

NOTES

Part 1
1. Larry Tye, "Patients At Risk: Hospital Errors," *Boston Globe* (14 March 1999).
2. Arthur L. Kellerman, "Deja Vu," *Annals of Emergency Medicine* 35 (January 2000): 83-85.1.
3. Robert Derlet and John Richards, "Overcrowding in the Nation's Emergency Departments: Complex Causes and Disturbing Effects," *Annals of Emergency Medicine* 35 (January 2000): 63-68.
4. Robert Derlet and John Richards, reply to letter to the editor, *Annals of Emergency Medicine* 36 (September 2000).
5. Derlet and Richards, "Overcrowding."
6. Robert Reinhold, "Crisis in Emergency Rooms: More Symptoms Than Cures," *Minnesota Medicine* 71 (November 1988): 688-91.
7. Derlet and Richards, "Overcrowding."
8. Andrew Bindman et. al., "Consequences of Queuing for Care at a Public Hospital Emergency Department," *Journal of the American Medical Association* 28 (August 1991): 1091-96.
9. David W. Baker et. al., "Patients Who Leave a Public Hospital Emergency Department Without Being Seen By a Physician: Causes and Consequences," *Journal of the American Medical Association* 28 (August 1991): 1085-90.

Part 2
1. Laura Johannes, "Clot Busters May Pose High Risks for Elderly," *Wall Street Journal* (May 8, 2000): sec. B2.
2. J. Lazarou et. al., "Incidence of Adverse Drug Reactions in Hospitalized Patients: a Meta-analysis of Prospective Studies," *Journal of the American Medical Association* 279 (1998): 1200-04.
3. J. Moore et. al., Commentary: "Time to act on drug safety," *Journal of the American Medical Association* 279 (May 1998): 1571-73.

4. T.B. Graboys et. al., "Results of a Second-Opinion Trial Among Patients Recommended for Coronary Angiography," *Journal of the American Medical Association 268* (Nov 1992): 2537-40.

5. L. Pilote et. al., "Differences in the Treatment of Myocardial Infarction in the United States and Canada," *Archives of Internal Medicine* (23 May 1994): 1090-96.

6. Jan Blustein, "High-Technology Cardiac Procedures. The Impact of Service Availability on Service Use in New York State," *Journal of the American Medical Association* (21 July 1993): 344-49.

7. Derlet and Richards, "Overcrowding."

8. M. F. Newman et. al., "Longitudinal Assessment of Neurocognitive Function after Coronary-Artery Bypass Surgery," *The New England Journal of Medicine* 344 (2001): 395-402.

9. E. S. Holmboel et. al., "Perceptions of Benefit and Risk of Patients Undergoing First-time Elective Percutaneous Coronary Revascularization," *Journal of General Internal Medicine* 15, 9: 632-637.

10. S. Selbst et. al., "Medication Errors in a Pediatric Emergency Department," *Pediatric Emergency Care* 15 (1999): 1-4.

11. R. Mehta and K. Eagle, "Missed Diagnosis of Acute Coronary Syndromes in the Emergency Room: Continuing Challenges," *The New England Journal of Medicine* 342 (2000): 1207-10.

12. E. J. Thomas and T. A. Brennan, "Incidence and Types of Preventable Adverse Events in Elderly Patients: Population Based Review of Medical Records," *British Medical Journal* 320 (2000): 741-44.

13. A. A. Gawande et. al., "The Incidence and Nature of Surgical Adverse Events in Colorado and Utah in 1992," *Surgery* 126 (1999): 66-75.

14. D.S. Rubasmen, "Jumping To Conclusions Costs Patients and Physicians," *Physician's Financial News* (28 February 2001).

15. S. A. Klein, "Evading an Emergency Call Can Put Doctors in Legal Peril," *American Medical News* (24 January 2000).

16. J. A. Ambrose and G. Dangas, "Unstable Angina: Current Concepts of Pathogenesis and Treatment," *Archives of Internal Medicine* 160 (2000): 25-37.

17. J. C. Brillman et. al., "Triage: Limitations in Predicting Need for Emergent Care and Hospital Admission," *Annals of Emergency Medicine* 27 (1996): 493-9.

18. Brian McCormick, "Most Doctors Say They Practice Defensive Medicine," *American Medical News* (25 May 1992).

19. Reynolds et. al., "The Cost of Medical Professional Liability," *Journal of the American Medical Association* 257 (1987): 2776-81.

20. "Doctors, Fearing Liability Suits, Resign," *Physician's Financial News* (1992): 47.

21. R. R. Roberts et. al., "Costs of an Emergency Department-Based Accelerated Diagnostic Protocol vs. Hospitalization in Patients With Chest Pain: A Randomized Controlled Trial," *Journal of the American Medical Association* 278 (1997): 1670-76.

22. D. Spurgeon and T.M. Burton, "For the Very Cautious, A Physical Exam Now Includes a CAT Scan," *Wall Street Journal* (23 March 2000): sec. A, p. 1, 12.

23. D. Alfaro et. al., "Accuracy of Interpretation of Cranial Computed Tomography Scans in an Emergency Medicine Residency Program," *Annals of Emergency Medicine*, (February 1995): 169-74.

24. H. R. Burstin et. al., "Socioeconomic Status and Risk for Substandard Medical Care," *Journal of the American Medical Association* (4 November 1992): 2383-87.

25. J. S. Weissman et. al., "Rates of Avoidable Hospitalization by Insurance Status in Massachusetts and Maryland," *Journal of the American Medical Association* (4 Nov 1992): 2388-94.

26. Ibid.

27. L. L. Leape et. al., "The Nature of Adverse Events in Hospitalized Patients: Results of the Harvard Medical Practice Study II," *New England Journal of Medicine* (1991): 377-84.

28. R. A. Dudley et. al., "Selective Referral to High-Volume Hospitals: Estimating Potentially Avoidable Deaths," *Journal of the American Medical Association* 283 (2000): 1159-66.

29. J. D. Birkmeyer, "High-Risk Surgery—Follow the Crowd," *Journal of the American Medical Association* 283 (1 March 2000): 1191-93.

30. J.G. Ouslander, "Inappropriate Hospitalization of Nursing Facility Residents: A Symptom of a Sick System of Care for Frail Older People," *Journal of the American Geriatric Society* 48 (February 2000): 230-231.

31. R.J. Ackerman, "Emergency Department Use by Nursing Home Residents," *Annals of Emergency Medicine* 31 (June 1998): 749-757.

32. Derlet and Richards, "Overcrowding."

33. Sheldon Jacobson, MD, "Avoidable Errors in Emergency Medicine," *Emergency Medicine* (January 1997).

Part 4

1. R.T. Cook, "The Institute of Medicine Report on Emergency Medical Services for Children: Thoughts for Emergency Medical Technicians, Paramedics and Emergency Physicians," *Pediatrics* 96 Supplement (1995): 199-210.

2. T.N. Raju et. al., "Medication Errors in Neonatal and Pediatric Intensive-Care Units," *Lancet* 2 (1989): 374-376.

3. H.L. Folli et. al., "Medication Error Prevention by Clinical Pharmacists in Two Children's Hospitals," *Pediatrics* 79 (1987): 718-722.

4. S.M. Selbst et. al., "Medication Errors in a Pediatric Emergency Department," *Pediatric Emergency Care* 15 (1999): 1-4.

5. Jerry Buckley, "The Shame of Emergency Care for Kids," *US News & World Report* (1992): 34-42.

6. P. W. Glaeser, et. al., "Survey of Nationally Registered Emergency Medical Services Providers: Pediatric Education," *Annals of Emergency Medicine* 36 (July 2000): 33-38.

7. "Pretty Poison," *Emergency Medicine* (30 June 1986): 69-82

INDEX

medication: allergic reactions to, 17, 31, 45; children, giving to, 167-172; proper dosages of, 170; errors, 44-45; side effects of, 45; stocking your medicine chest, 186-189; Web sites, 189
migraine, 151
misdiagnosis, avoiding, 43
MRI, 27

N

nausea, 130, 132, 134, 140, 141, 143, 151, 167. *See also* vomiting
neglect. *See* delays, treatment
New England Journal of Medicine, 30
nurse practitioner, 63

O

older adults, 29-30, 43; abdominal pain in, 140; appendicitis in, 51, 144-145; diabetes in, 132; heart attack in, 16, 34, 131-132, misdiagnosis in, 132; hospitalization risks for, 105; stroke risk in, 133-135; Web sites, 101, 189
overcrowding, 1, 2, 7-11, 41, 109, 110; causes of, 8-11; consequences of, 2, 26, 29; definition of, 7, 8

P

pain: prolonged, 30; types of, 140-141
paronychia, 24, 25
patient advocate: hospital appointed, 44, 122; need for, 35-36, 41, 42
pediatrics. *See* children
pelvic inflammatory disease, 141
penicillin, 17
Physician's Desk Reference, 18, 45, 140
"physician-phobia", 108
physician's assistant, 63

pill-popping, 16
planning ahead, xi, xii, 2, 42, 117, 126; for end-of-life decisions, 99-100; tips on, 42
Poison Control, 166; Web site, 174
poisoning, 74; in children, 164-166
Power of Attorney, *see* health-care proxy
prescription drugs; adverse reactions to, 17; legible handwriting by doctor, 44; pulled from market, 17
procedures, medical: commonly performed, 21-25; questions to ask about, 31-32; risks of, 20, 21; unnecessary, 19-21, 77
Professional Standard, The, 33
pulmonary embolism, 133

R

resistant bacteria. *See* drug resistance
Reye's syndrome, 169, 172
"RICE", 146
ripped off at the ER register, 118-123; how to avoid being, 121-123
risk vs. benefit approach, 20, 30-34, 52

S

second opinion, importance of, 56
seizure, and fever, 153
"service patient", 88, 91
shortness of breath, 137-138
specialists, 48-50; alternatives to ER, 179; delays, caused by, 49, 50, 52, 53; incompetence of, 48, 49, 52; solving the dilemma of, 54-56; tips for getting quality care from, 54-56; types of, 184-185
staff, ER, 59-63, 70, 183; shortages/cuts, 11

stroke, 133-137; in older adults, 133-135; clot dissolving treatment for, 136-137; risk factors of, 134-136; symptoms of, 133-134; treatment delays, 26-28, 38, 136; two types, 27-28, 133-134; Web sites, 39, 137
sudden illness, guidelines, 125-126

T

Ten Commandments of the ER, 126-128
tests: commonly performed, 21; imperfect, 81-83; inaccurate, 82, 83; misinterpreted results, 84; questions to ask about, 31-32, 85-86; putting too much trust in, 81; unnecessary, 18, 35; useless, 83, 84
Tetanus shot, 147
three day rule, 127-128
torsion, 141
tPA treatment, 15, 22-23, 136-137
Transient Ischemic Attack (TIA), 135
treatments: delays in, 25-29, 35, 36-38, 49, 50, 53; risky/unnecessary, 18, 35, 42; tips to reduce risks of, 34-35; worse than disease, 15, 19
triage, 70-75; definition of, 70; errors in, 71; tips to avoid errors in, 72-75; travesties in, 70

U

uninsured. *See* "service patient"
urgent care facility, 176-177
U.S. News and World Report, 95, 158

V

visceral pain, 141
vomiting, 74, 130, 134, 140,

ABOUT THE AUTHOR

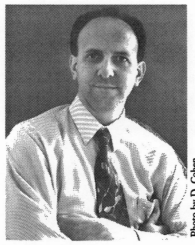

Photo by D. Cohen

Joel Cohen, MD has practiced emergency and urgent care medicine for nearly a decade. He is a former Clinical Instructor of Medicine at New York University School of Medicine and a former Clinical Assistant Professor at New York University School of Nursing. Dr. Cohen writes about health topics for cbshealthwatch.com and other Web sites. He lives in New York with his family.

For more information about emergency care log on to:
http://www.emergencyhealth.com.